Memory and Attention Adaptation Training

Memory and Attention Adaptation Training

A Brief Cognitive Behavioral Therapy for Cancer Survivors

Survivor Workbook

Robert J. Ferguson, PhD

Assistant Professor of Medicine, Department of Medicine

Division of Hematology/Oncology

University of Pittsburgh School of Medicine and

UPMC Hillman Cancer Center

Pittsburgh, PA, USA

Karen Lee Gillock, PhD

Licensed Clinical Psychologist

Cognitive-Behavioral Therapy

Lebanon, NH, USA

OXFORD

UNIVERSITY PRESS

OXFORD
UNIVERSITY PRESS

Oxford University Press is a department of the University of Oxford. It furthers the University's objective of excellence in research, scholarship, and education by publishing worldwide. Oxford is a registered trade mark of Oxford University Press in the UK and certain other countries.

Published in the United States of America by Oxford University Press
198 Madison Avenue, New York, NY 10016, United States of America.

ISBN 978–0–19–752152–6

DOI: 10.1093/med/9780197521526.001.0001

This material is not intended to be, and should not be considered, a substitute for medical or other professional advice. Treatment for the conditions described in this material is highly dependent on the individual circumstances. And, while this material is designed to offer accurate information with respect to the subject matter covered and to be current as of the time it was written, research and knowledge about medical and health issues is constantly evolving and dose schedules for medications are being revised continually, with new side effects recognized and accounted for regularly. Readers must therefore always check the product information and clinical procedures with the most up-to-date published product information and data sheets provided by the manufacturers and the most recent codes of conduct and safety regulation. The publisher and the authors make no representations or warranties to readers, express or implied, as to the accuracy or completeness of this material. Without limiting the foregoing, the publisher and the authors make no representations or warranties as to the accuracy or efficacy of the drug dosages mentioned in the material. The authors and the publisher do not accept, and expressly disclaim, any responsibility for any liability, loss, or risk that may be claimed or incurred as a consequence of the use and/or application of any of the contents of this material.

1 3 5 7 9 8 6 4 2

Printed by Integrated Books International, United States of America

Contents

Acknowledgments

MAAT cancer survivor research was funded by grants from the National Cancer Institute (R03 CA90151; R-21CA143619), the Lance Armstrong Foundation, and The Beckwith Institute, Pittsburgh, PA, and ongoing research with a grant funded by the National Cancer Institute (R01CA244673). MAAT traumatic brain injury research was funded by the Eunice Kennedy Shriver National Institute of Child Health and Human Development of the National Institutes of Health (R01 HD047242).

We want to express deep gratitude to all research participants and their families for devoting valuable time to MAAT research. Without participants, there can be no research on this treatment program or others in cancer care and thus no knowledge gained. Thank you.

We also wish to thank all cancer survivors who have undergone MAAT in numerous clinical practices in both the United States and other countries and have provided valuable feedback for making improvements in the usability of MAAT.

About This Program

At the time of this writing, approximately 16 million American men and women are cancer survivors.[1] According to the National Cancer Institute, the term "survivor" includes any individual who has ever been given a diagnosis of cancer. Because of a combination of increased awareness of cancer, widespread screening, early detection technologies, and improved treatments, more people are living longer and fuller lives after a cancer diagnosis than at any other time in history. In fact, the number of cancer deaths has been in steady decline since 1991, which is good news after decades of growing numbers of deaths caused by cancer. Cancer deaths dropped by 2.2% from 2016 to 2017, the largest single-year drop in cancer mortality ever recorded.[2] From this perspective, there is much to celebrate in the health care battle against cancer.

Despite this good news, cancer remains a formidable challenge for patients, families, employers, health care professionals, and communities. Once cancer is detected, the treatments are often complex, and decision-making about the best treatment options is far from simple. Many cancer treatments give rise to significant side effects that are disruptive to work and family life. For example, each year in the United States, over 1 million Americans undergo chemotherapy to treat many different types of cancer. The process of chemotherapy can often be arduous and many patients can experience side effects such as fatigue, nausea, and nerve-related pain experienced as tingling pain in fingers and toes (also known as peripheral neuropathy). For the most part, these symptoms improve after chemotherapy has been completed. However, some symptoms persist beyond chemotherapy. Other treatments, such hormone suppression therapies for prostate or breast cancer, or certain immune therapies, can lead to side effects that may persist well after treatment stops. Disruptions in cognitive functions of memory and attention have gained considerable attention over the past 30 years related to cancer and cancer treatment, and these are the target of this program.

Research has shown that roughly half of the individuals who have been diagnosed with and treated for cancer may complain of persistent memory and attention problems such as slowed thinking and not being able to recall words or follow conversations. In the past this has been called "chemobrain" or "chemofog," but research has shown that cancer itself—even if the cancer is not in the brain but in other parts of the body—may produce problems with memory. The term currently used is "cancer-related cognitive impairment," or CRCI. While most people with cancer may report memory problems during active treatment, a subgroup of individuals have been observed to have CRCI for much longer—up to 2, 5, or even more years after treatment. These memory and attention problems are usually not severe but rather fall in a mild to moderate range. Nevertheless, they can be frustrating to experience, can disrupt job tasks or career goals, disturb social and family relationships, and interfere with an active and healthy life.

This program—Memory and Attention Adaptation Training (MAAT)—is for cancer survivors who have memory and attention complaints or CRCI associated with their cancer experience. CRCI problems may arise from:

- Cancer of the brain and central nervous system; problems with attention and memory that can be due to cancer itself;
- Surgery to remove brain tumors or other cancer-related surgery of the brain;
- Intrathecal therapies (anti-cancer or other drugs delivered into the spinal fluid);
- Radiation therapy such as whole-body radiation therapy or cranial radiation therapies (either targeting a region in the brain or whole-brain radiation);
- Hormonal therapies such as selective estrogen receptor modulator (SERM) drugs (e.g., tamoxifen) or aromatase inhibiting

drugs, or AIs (e.g., anastrozole [Arimidex] or exemestane [Aromasin]);
- Androgen therapies used to treat prostate cancer;
- Stem cell transplant (chemotherapy followed by transplant of early blood cells, or "stem cells," from the blood stream); and/or
- Autologous (within the same person) or allogeneic (from a donor) bone marrow transplant (chemotherapy, followed by transplant of early blood cells from bone marrow).

Because of the large number of people experiencing cancer-related memory problems, it only makes sense to apply current knowledge to help cancer survivors better manage the impact of memory problems in daily life. Many scientific questions remain as to just how cancer treatments affect memory and attention function. However, as we await results of ongoing research, the point of MAAT is to use existing cognitive-behavioral technologies and strategies that are known to have a positive impact on cancer survivors' quality of life and performance on tasks that require good attention and memory skills.

MAAT is a brief cognitive-behavioral therapy that uses behavioral and cognitive strategies shown in research to help people cope with and self-manage problems of memory and attention in everyday life. MAAT will not help you gain a "photographic memory" or promise supernatural memory power. There are any manner of products, natural supplements, computer-assistive devices, computer training programs, and workshops on the market that can aid memory and attention. However, often these approaches do not live up to their claims or are not targeted to people who have gone through cancer treatment. MAAT is a bit different. It is specifically designed to help you learn behavioral compensatory skills to better manage CRCI problems in real-world daily activity. It is also designed to be practical so you can adapt and cope with the numerous stress demands that may be harder to meet after cancer. We believe MAAT will be most useful and practical for you by helping you learn and adapt strategies suited to your own circumstances (this is why the word *Adaptation* is in the title).

There are four parts to MAAT:

1. *Education and reattribution*: This covers how memory and attention works and reviews how these abilities are affected by chemotherapy or other cancer treatments. It also covers how other factors, such as genetic influences or everyday stress, affect memory.
2. *Self-awareness training*: This refers to observing your own memory and attention behavior and identifying the type and nature of memory problems you experience. By knowing the factors that affect your memory and attention, such as environment (e.g., noise, visual distractions), emotions, and physical states (e.g., fatigue), you can target these variables to prevent or change them.
3. *Stress management skills*: This involves developing strategies, such as relaxation, to help manage stress, which can make memory and attention problems worse, and to enhance general coping.
4. *Compensatory strategies*: These techniques are designed to help prevent or reduce memory and attention failures in daily life and improve personal performance at family, social, work, or recreational activities. They are adapted from research on treatment of memory and attention problems in behavior therapy and cognitive rehabilitation.

MAAT involves eight visits of around 45 to 60 minutes each and can be done individually with a psychologist (or other health professional) or in small groups. Like most cognitive-behavioral therapies, MAAT is goal-focused and time-limited. In each visit you will learn skills to practice at home between visits. The point of practice is the practical application of strategies in everyday, real-life situations. The strategies can be modified so they best suit you and your life. It is the philosophy of MAAT that memory and attention skills are of little use if they are not practical or simple to apply. Your clinician will take the time in each visit to review the application of strategies, deal with problems of applying strategies, and identify modifications so they are useful. You will find that no, you are not crazy, and no, you are not imagining attention and memory lapses during and after cancer and cancer treatment. This support alone sometimes enhances coping and resilience. You will also devise a plan to help you keep up your new memory and attention skills so that you will maintain them—always. The schedule for the program is seen in Table 1.1 of the Visit 1 section of this workbook.

Are You Ready For MAAT?

MAAT is a program of cognitive and behavioral changes that requires time and practice to achieve maximum benefit. Research on cancer survivorship and plain experience tells us that the diagnosis of cancer brings all sorts of stresses. These include treatment decisions, disruptions to family life and social relationships, work disruptions, costs for health care and financial worries, and juggling a busy schedule. Further, cancer is often not the only chronic health problem some cancer survivors must pay attention to and self-manage. Other chronic illnesses such as diabetes, high blood pressure, heart disease, asthma, or neurologic problems (stroke or movement disorders) can coexist with cancer. It is little wonder that psychologists with health psychology or behavioral medicine training are enlisted to help patients and families make the best adaptations they can in living with these conditions.

MAAT is intended for cancer survivors who have completed cancer treatments or are nearing the end of their treatment. The reason for this is to avoid adding more appointments to the already busy schedule of the person with cancer. For individuals with difficult-to-control depression, severe anxiety, or other psychiatric illness, we recommend addressing that before starting MAAT. In addition, we recommend addressing any problems with alcohol or other substance use or addiction problems and ensuring these conditions are well managed before starting MAAT. For individuals who may have severe memory impairment due to cancer involving the brain or who have had other neurologic complications such as a stroke or seizures, we recommend getting a thorough evaluation by a neurologist and getting neuropsychological testing by a licensed neuropsychologist. The only objective way to measure memory function is with standard neuropsychological tests, and a licensed neuropsychologist is the expert who can do this.

Finally, if you question whether you are ready for this program and are not sure of your motivation, simply take this workbook home and read it over. Don't feel obligated to complete any of the exercises or learn the strategies; rather, review it at your own pace. See what you can expect from it and if it would benefit you. After this, let your clinician know what you would like to do.

That being said, getting started with MAAT may never come at a perfect time. As the old adage says, "If not now, when?" Below are some questions to consider before starting MAAT:

1. Do I have memory or attention problems that interfere with my family activities, work, and social life?
2. Do others point out to me or show concern (either verbally or nonverbally) that I have forgotten a conversation or information just told me?
3. Do I have the time now to devote to the weekly or near-weekly MAAT visits?
4. Can I ask family members, friends, co-workers, or community members to help me with transportation to MAAT visits or set aside time for video visits (e.g., help with responsibilities, leave work early to get to appointments)?
5. Do I believe MAAT can help improve my function and quality of life?

In all likelihood, if you answered yes to three out of these five questions, you are ready to begin.

Visit 1

In This Visit You Will:

- Complete the introduction to MAAT and go over the schedule in Table 1.1.
- Review memory and attention and problems associated with cancer.
- Review how self-awareness can improve memory performance.
- Learn how to self-monitor memory and attention failures so that you can anticipate problem situations and choose the most effective strategies.
- Learn about and practice Progressive Muscle Relaxation.

MAAT

The name of this program, Memory and Attention Adaptation Training (MAAT), emphasizes *adaptation.* Our aim is to have you start adapting new ways of doing things you did before cancer and cancer treatment in order to minimize the effects of ongoing memory problems. You are certainly not alone in survivorship. As of 2016, there were 15.5 million cancer survivors in the United States alone, with the number projected to grow to about 20.3 million by 2026.[1,2] So problems with memory and attention related to cancer affects many, and we hope MAAT will be of help to you. MAAT involves eight visits, each about 45-50 minutes long, once per week. The content of each visit is outlined in Table 1.1. This may vary depending on your speed and what is practical for you. You will use this workbook to guide you through the program step by step, so be sure to bring it with you to each MAAT visit. Feel free to underline or highlight parts of the text you believe are important.

Table 1.1 MAAT Schedule

Visit	Content
1	• Introduction and MAAT overview • Education on memory and attention and effects of cancer and treatment • Memory failure reattribution: Not all memory failures are cancer-related • Self-awareness and monitoring memory problems • Progressive muscle relaxation • Homework
2	• Review MAAT reading, relaxation and quick relaxation review, rehearsal • Review self-monitoring, effects of context, senses and memory problems • Internal strategy: Self-Instructional Training (SIT) • Homework
3	• Quick relaxation review • Review application of SIT • Internal strategy: verbal rehearsal strategies (verbal rehearsal, spaced rehearsal, chunking, and rhymes) • Cognitive restructuring: realistic probabilities and decatastrophizing • Homework
4	• Review of verbal rehearsal strategies • Review realistic probabilities and decatastrophizing • External strategy: keeping a schedule and memory routines • Homework
5	• Review of keeping a schedule and memory routines • External strategies: external cueing and distraction reduction • Activity scheduling and pacing • Homework
6	• Review of external cueing, distraction reduction, and activity scheduling and pacing • Internal and external strategy: active listening, verbal rehearsal for socializing • Fatigue management and sleep improvement • Homework
7	• Review active listening, verbal rehearsal for socializing • Review fatigue management and sleep quality improvement • Internal strategy: visualization strategies • Homework
8	• Review visualization strategies • Tying it together and continued quality-of-life improvement in survivorship • Discussion and wrap-up

Review of Memory and Attention Problems Associated with Cancer

The types of memory and attention problems many cancer survivors report differ among individuals and also depend on type of cancer treatment received. In this section, we will review the various memory problems that have been reported in research on cancer-related cognitive impairments (CRCI) with a general overview. Be sure to ask your clinician to clarify anything you have questions about or direct you to a reliable source of information on CRCI.

Common memory problems associated with CRCI may include inability to recall specific words or phrases just heard or read a short time before; forgetting names or phone numbers; and difficulty paying attention while taking steps through tasks and procedures (for example, steps in cooking or mechanical repair tasks). However, these problems vary from person to person. Some people report no problems with memory or attention after cancer. Others find they have entirely different problems of memory or attention, such as word finding difficulty. Typical memory and attention problems cancer survivors report after cancer are outlined in Table 1.2. These problems were identified in research on cancer patients who have undergone chemotherapy, but you may or may not find your experience matches this list. Many of these same symptoms have been reported by individuals who have undergone other forms of treatment, including hormonal therapies (endocrine therapies such as tamoxifen), radiation therapy, or surgery.

As you can see, survivors report a wide range of memory and attention problems. For example, in one scientific report that reviewed 16 different studies on memory effects of chemotherapy, the range of detected memory problems in the study varied from 0% to 75%! Overall, it is believed that roughly a quarter to about half of all people who have been diagnosed with and treated for cancer may have some decline in memory and attention abilities when objectively measured by standardized memory tests. Part of the reason for the large disagreements between the studies has to do with the fact that

Table 1.2 Common Attention and Memory Problems Reported by Cancer Survivors

1. Recalling names
2. Recalling things when trying hard
3. Recalling written details on a form
4. Recalling written information or things viewed on television
5. Remembering names, faces of people recently met
6. Making sense out of verbal explanations
7. Recalling what happened just a few minutes ago
8. Paying attention to what is going on in the immediate environment
9. Following what people are saying
10. Staying alert to what is going on

the researchers used different tests. Other reasons may be due to different effects of different cancers or different treatments. Regardless, the bottom line is that a large segment of cancer survivors experience memory problems. In the vast majority of cases they appear to be mild or moderate, but many survivors report that the problems disrupt daily life, as seen in Table 1.2.

Many cancer survivors report that their CRCI symptoms had a gradual onset. For example, an older survey completed by Hurricane Voices Breast Cancer Foundation revealed that 79% of the 471 patients said their symptoms came on gradually rather than suddenly. So this gradual onset of memory problems may be fairly common. About half of survivors reported that their symptoms "come and go," while the other half reported that they are "always present." Again, there is variability in the nature of the memory problems. Finally, 23% of survey respondents reported they had completed cancer treatment five years prior to taking the survey. Of these, 92% reported persistent problems with memory. So for some individuals with CRCI, the memory problems are long-lasting.

While we know that many cancer survivors will report memory and attention problems after receiving various forms of cancer and cancer therapy, it is not fully known why some people may experience CRCI and others may not. Moreover, there is some variability in the experience of CRCI. For instance, past studies suggest that high-dose chemotherapy may have a greater negative effect on memory. Still other research implies that reducing estrogen activity (a hormone associated with breast cancer *and* memory function) may play a role in negatively affecting attention and memory through causing a reduction in estrogen availability (for example, medicines such as Tamoxifen that block the actions of estrogen, or aromatase inhibiting medicines that block the production of estrogen, such as Arimidex). However, men naturally produce less estrogen than women but also report memory problems after chemotherapy or other cancer treatments, so estrogen reduction alone may not fully explain CRCI.

Genetic factors that may have a role in CRCI continue to be studied. One genetic marker, apolipoprotein E (APOE), appears to make some people vulnerable to memory problems after mild traumatic brain injury (or concussion) or the oxygen reduction effects of open heart surgery. People who have this genetic characteristic may also be more vulnerable to memory problems after chemotherapy. However, in recent research APOE did not appear to have much of an influence on memory function. This result is not final, as it may be that certain types of chemotherapy, radiation therapy, immunotherapy, or other treatments may affect APOE-positive individuals more than others. Further, more genetic factors may be at play with APOE in a complex interaction of factors, making the "genetic vulnerability" question a difficult one to answer.

There is a question about how chemotherapy or other things (such as injury) may change brain circuitry and how the cerebral cortex functions. The cerebral cortex is the large, outer portion of the brain largely responsible for associative learning, reasoning, and goal-directed behavior, which uses all forms of memory. One study conducted by the first author and colleagues at Dartmouth Medical School studied these possible effects in 60-year-old women who were identical twins. Because they were identical, they shared the exact same genetic makeup, and both were APOE positive. One was diagnosed and treated with chemotherapy and hormonal therapy for breast cancer; the other did not have breast cancer or any cancer treatment. Each was asked to complete a small battery of neuropsychological tests of memory and also complete a cognitive task in an MRI scanner—known as "functional MRI (fMRI)." The task they

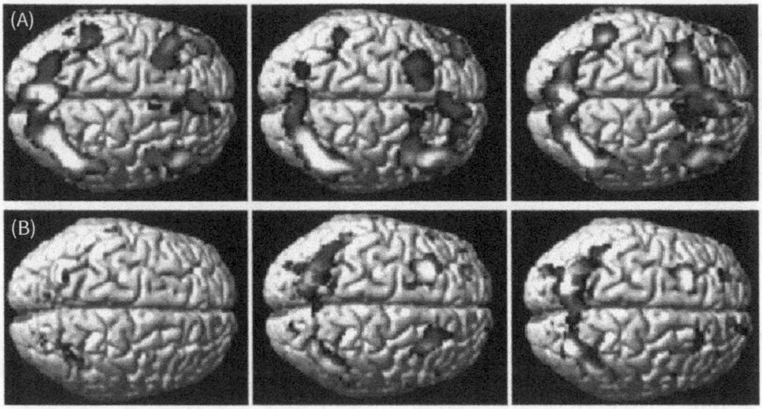

Figure 1.1 fMRI images of twins doing a memory task that gets more difficult from left to right. Note that the twin who received chemotherapy (**A**) appears to have more activation of the brain for the same task than her non-cancer twin (**B**).

completed was a visual memory task that gets more difficult over three phases. Figure 1.1 displays images of each of the twins' brains.

Going left to right, the task gets more difficult. As shown, the shaded and darker areas indicate more activity in the cortex (measured as blood flow). The brain image on top is the twin who had chemotherapy (**A**); on the bottom is the non-cancer twin (**B**). As seen, the twin who had chemotherapy shows much greater activity in the cortex both at the simplest level of the task and at more difficult levels (moving right) than her sister. Of course, the unaffected twin (**B**) also shows more activity as the task gets more difficult from left to right, but far less than her sister who had cancer treatment.

Interestingly, each twin performed about the same on the task in the scanner and on the neuropsychological memory tests. The one difference between them was that the twin who had chemotherapy reported more difficulty with daily memory problems or symptoms than her unaffected twin. The conclusion of this twin study? Well, we cannot be certain, but the fact that there was more activation in the survivor's cortex while performing at the same level as her "normal" sister suggests that the breast cancer survivor's cortex is compensating for damaged associative memory circuits by "rewiring" or using more alternative circuits. That is, more brain is used to complete the same level of task performance. This might explain why many people who have undergone chemotherapy or other cancer treatments may score normally on standardized neuropsychological memory tests, but report they are different or slower, or that they "have to work harder to get the same result" when using their memory.

While research continues to use brain imaging methods, larger studies using multiple survivors have reached findings similar to the twin study.[3,4] The collection of these findings implies that the brain recovers after injury and can "rewire" new circuits to help with recovery of daily task performance.

Other factors that can negatively affect memory and attention after chemotherapy include the effects of anxiety, stress, and depressed mood. To be clear, the effects of cancer treatments such as chemotherapy are NOT solely due to these factors, so you can rest assured we are not saying that "chemofog" or CRCI is due to stress or anxiety. Past research has controlled for anxiety, stress and depressive symptoms and still we see memory performance scores that are lower in chemotherapy than non-chemotherapy cancer survivors.

Nevertheless, the impact of stress and anxiety on memory and attention function is profound. When people are stressed, anxious or have depressive symptoms, there are significant physical changes in the body that include respiration, blood flow in areas of the brain, other organs and muscles, and overall muscle tension. These responses happen to everyone under normal everyday conditions and in times of high stress. They serve the important function of helping the body deal with demands placed on it, whether these demands are from family, work, illness, or some immediate physical threat such as a wild animal attack. Basically, what the brain is trying to do is to help redirect blood, which is rich in oxygen and nutrients, to muscles in the body and critical areas of the brain—but the "thinking areas" of the brain have reduced blood flow. In someone with chronic anxiety or depressed mood (anxiety and depression that go on for a long time), the resulting changes can lead to decreased ability to focus and trouble paying attention. In turn, this interferes with the process of encoding or storing information to later be recalled as a memory. That is, problems remembering can result from information that has not been properly "stored" to begin with. Therefore, anxiety, stress and mood can negatively affect memory and attention.

Certainly, managing these problems has been studied and successful behavioral and cognitive therapies have been developed and shown to be effective in mitigating stress effects on the brain and body. While we may not fully understand the effects of the various cancer treatments on memory and attention function, we *do* know the effects of stress. This is true for everyone whether they are a cancer survivor who as undergone extensive treatment or not.

The Point of MAAT: Improve What We Know We Can

An important point needs to be made here. After reading this far, you might be wondering, "well if we know so little about this problem, how are we going to solve it?" Or, perhaps even more cynically, "why even bother?" Here is the point of MAAT: Let's focus on what is known.

We do know:

1) Various forms of cancer and cancer treatment can lead to long-term attention and memory problems for many cancer survivors.
2) These problems appear to be subtle but appear to be most bothersome for people when they begin to resume more demanding levels of work, family, and recreational activity after cancer therapy has ended.
3) These same types of problems may occur during or after other cancer treatments, such as endocrine or hormonal therapies, bone marrow transplant, surgery, or radiation treatments, or

perhaps the cancer itself. More research on all these areas is ongoing.

4) Stress, anxiety, and depression do not appear to be the sole causes of memory problems after cancer treatment. However, stress, anxiety, and depressed mood, though not a direct *cause* of memory problems, can still *contribute* and *add* to problems.
5) Often, individuals who are aware of trouble with memory and attention are understandably concerned. This concern can raise worry, and then raise the stress response. Therefore, a cycle of worry and stress can make the memory problems worse.

What we do know is how to manage the impact of memory problems on daily life *and* how to manage stress in busy 21st century life. This is what MAAT aims to help you do.

It is also important to understand that people who are healthy and who have never had any brain injury, neurological disease, or other medical conditions affecting the brain also report frequent problems with memory or attention. Indeed, often! By keeping this in mind, not *every* instance of forgetting a name, or forgetting what was spoken about in a meeting, or trouble thinking is an indication of memory disturbance. Ironically, "forgetting" actually serves an important survival function—it is the brain's way of sorting out the important from the unimportant and keeping "mental clutter" to a minimum. There is a condition called "hyperthymesia" which is characterized by being able to remember every life event in vivid detail. This is exceedingly rare, but of the few individuals with this condition, some report problems of not being able to "move on" from painful or embarrassing memories. In a sense, there is too much mental clutter getting in the way of living moment to moment.

Table 1.3 lists daily memory and attention problems reported by healthy adults. To the right of the list is the percentage of people who report experiencing the problem.

As seen, reports of different types of episodes of forgetfulness are common. *The point here is this*: if one jumps to the conclusion that

Table 1.3 Common Things People Forget

Problem	Percent of People
Forgets telephone numbers	58%
Forgets people's names	48%
Forgets where car was parked	32%
Loses car keys	31%
Forgets groceries	28%
Forgets why they entered a room	27%
Forgets directions	24%
Forgets appointment dates	20%
Forgets store locations in shopping center	20%
Loses items around the house	17%
Loses wallet or pocketbook	17%
Forgets content of daily conversations	17%

* Source: Mittenberg W, Zielinski R, Fichera S. Recovery from mild head injury: A treatment manual for patients. *Psychotherapy in Private Practice* 1993;12:37–52.

every lapse in memory or attention is due to something wrong with the brain, it may only add to stress, which will indeed add to attention and memory trouble. That is, not every memory or attention lapse is completely attributable to chemotherapy or other forms of cancer treatment. Therefore, to stop this vicious cycle, keep in mind Table 1.3 and the fact that minor memory and attention problems are part of everyday healthy living. Yes, they occur in conjunction with CRCI, but cancer treatment may not be the culprit of all problems of forgetting or trouble paying attention.

To summarize:

1) We know that cancer and cancer treatment can produce problems in memory and attention. This may not be the case with every cancer survivor but those that report problems may have them for a long time.
2) At present it is not known exactly how chemotherapy or other treatments affect memory and attention function. We do know

that other common factors, such as daily stress and the effects of anxiety and depression can adversely affect paying attention and remembering.

3) Keep in mind not all memory failures in daily life will be attributable to chemotherapy or cancer treatment. Some will be, but these other factors can contribute to memory failures. So, controlling what we can, such as stress reactions, being mindful by paying attention and "remembering to remember" is key.
4) In the mean time, our attempt here is to use what knowledge we have available from behavioral research to help people *cope* with and *self-manage* memory and attention problems as research continues identifying neurological processes of the problem. By focusing our energies on what we do know, and applying behavior change and memory management strategies we know can help people cope and feel more confident, the first steps can be taken to improve quality of life and management of memory problems in cancer survivorship. That is the focus of MAAT.

Types of Memory and Attention

The first part of any program that addresses problems of memory and attention involves learning more about these functions. Being familiar with different types of memory and attention can help identify your particular strengths and weaknesses and help plan strategies that play up *your* particular strengths. No one has perfect memory or is perfectly attentive all the time. In fact, one news story highlights this fact. Joshua Foer, a freelance journalist, had heard about memory championships where contestants compete at tasks such as who can be the fastest at remembering the order of a shuffled deck of cards or remembering the longest sequence of random numbers. Not only did he investigate the United States Memory Championships, but he also actually entered, trained, and set a record! However, even though he trained his memory to almost superhuman heights for competitive tasks, he still has memory failures in everyday living.

"The sad truth is, I still forget where I parked my car all the time," he said in an interview with National Public Radio on February 23, 2011. "I still forget why it was that I opened the refrigerator door. I still forget to put down the toilet seat."

In summary, the strategies used to enhance memory function need to be applied to everyday life, *where memory is used.* As Mr. Foer says, "The thing about these techniques is they only work if you remember to use them. That's sort of the funny thing. You've got to remember to remember." (You can hear or read this interview archived at www.npr.org.) Knowing some basics of memory and attention can help you understand why failures in daily life such as these occur, even in memory "champions."

Attention is not just one concept of human awareness but involves some fundamental systems. Basic forms of *attention* include the following:

1) *Orientation attention*—The purpose of this form of attention is to alert us to something important; maybe a danger, a source of food, or a new and interesting object in the environment. We use orientation when we look to see where a loud noise came from.
2) *Sustained attention*—This type of attention keeps us focused on a task such as reading or listening to a teacher.
3) *Divided attention*—This form of attention enables us to split our attention for doing two things at once, such as driving while talking.
4) *Shifting attention*—This is the type of attention that lets us go from one task to another, such as stirring a pot while cooking, reading a recipe, then measuring and adding salt to the pot.

Attention is critical to *encoding.* Encoding is the process of putting new information into memory storage so that the new information can be learned and used either to carry out a task or to add to one's general knowledge. MAAT emphasizes mindfulness and attentiveness to the immediate learning task. Divided attention and distraction can detract from the process of attention and lead to reduced encoding. Since the advent of the smartphone and tablet, along with other mobile devices, the numerous distractions and interruptions these devices pose can have a detrimental effect on memory encoding. More of this is discussed in the section on distraction reduction.

As with attention, memory functions are divided among some basic systems. There are extensive writings and research on many forms of memory function that are not listed here. To help with memory in everyday life, we don't need to delve into the depths of the topic. However, here are some of the basic *memory* functions:

1) *Short-term memory*—This is memory that helps us recall things we just heard, saw, or read (within the past few minutes). An example is recalling a name of a person you just met a few minutes ago. This may also be called short-term *recall*.
2) *Long-term memory*—This is memory that allows you to remember significant things from long ago, such as a childhood memory, or things learned from a half-hour to an hour ago. This is also called long-term *recall*. A version of this that involves remembering facts, such as the date of birth of a grandparent or a historical event, is *declarative memory*.
3) *Working memory*—This is memory that allows you to hold information in your mind so you can use it to perform some act, such as going into another room to get something, or tell someone a phone number, or hearing a ZIP code and then writing it down. Working memory also helps us to remember the steps in a task, such as tying a shoe, building a birdhouse, or cooking.
4) *Recognition*—This type of memory helps you recognize things you might have forgotten; then, when you see them, you remember. A good example is when you go grocery shopping but forgot the list. At the store, you remember the items on the list because the things on the shelves remind you of items you may want. Recognition is usually easier than recall.

Again, it is not important to know these types of attention and memory functions inside and out. This is your workbook, and you can turn to this section anytime this topic comes to mind and you have a question. It is helpful to understand the basics of memory and attention systems. We know from research on the cognitive effects of cancer that many survivors report difficulty with short-term memory, working memory, recall, shifting, and divided attention. Good examples of these are listed in the prior list and in Table 1.2.

Memory and Attention Adaptation Skills

Self-Awareness and Monitoring Memory Problems

The first step in learning strategies to help aid memory and attention is to look more closely at when, where, and under what circumstances you experience memory and attention problems. As the title of this section implies, being more aware of factors that affect your memory and attention can help you prepare and do something about your memory function. Tiredness, stress, noise, emotions, and even hunger can affect memory and attention. For example, emotion can enhance memory and deepen the "network" of interconnected brain cells that store the memory. Think of where you were when you first heard the news of the attacks on New York, Washington DC, and Pennsylvania on September 11, 2001. Most people can recall what they were doing, whom they were with, and what room they were in. By contrast, try to recall what you had for lunch last Tuesday or the name of a medication you saw in an advertisement online or on television last evening. Because this probably has less emotional impact, you probably don't remember it.

Similar to emotion, the sensory systems used in establishing a memory can influence how well the memory is processed, stored, and then recalled. For example, some people, such as painters, photographers, or interior designers, are "visual." They may have an easier time picturing concepts in their minds or may remember visual features of something easier than its sound. Others are better at learning concepts with words they hear or the sounds produced by something they want to remember (such as remembering a bird species by its call rather than its appearance). Still others prefer to learn and remember things that are written, and others may remember by touch—such as the feeling of a sea shell, the wooden handle of a tool, or the texture of bread dough. Whether it is information that is seen, read, felt, or heard, the sensory system you use most will influence your attention and memory.

Keeping a brief record or "diary" of your memory and attention problems can help you discover variables that can influence them, such as emotional impact and sensory impact. Again, once you become aware of the circumstances affecting your memory and attention, you can make plans and learn skills that target your specific types of memory and attention problems. You may ask, "I already know when my memory or attention problems come up, so why should I keep a record of when this happens?" It is true that in many cases it's clear what situations can lead to trouble remembering. However, as with so much of human behavior, things that trigger problems of memory or attention may happen outside our awareness. The problems may be subtle and may differ depending on the situation. For example, some people may have trouble remembering conversations at work meetings with multiple participants but have less difficulty in social situations where they are more relaxed or with fewer people.

Form 1.1 is a memory and attention problem record. Feel free to make as many copies of this form as necessary. You should complete one record for only those memory and attention problems that bother you—those that have interfered with your work, leisure, or family life. You do not have to complete one record for each time you had trouble remembering or paying attention—that is unrealistic. But do try to sit down at least once a day and think back to situations where you had trouble remembering or paying attention. If you can, it is even better to complete one of these records as soon as possible after the problem. This helps with accuracy of details. A completed example of a record is also shown in Form 1.1.

Once you have filled out several of these forms, you can review them and look for patterns. For instance, are you having difficulty with short-term memory mostly for verbal-auditory information

Form 1.1 Memory and Attention Problem Record

Memory and Attention Problem Record

Date:_________________________ Time: ____________AM PM

How much did the memory or attention problem bother you?

0	1	2	3	4	5	6	7	8	9	10
Not at all				Moderately						Extremely

What the memory or attention problem was:

What was happening (where you were, what you were doing, and what the surroundings were like, e.g., noisy, quiet, etc.)

What I felt at the time (Anxious? Tense? Hungry? Tired? Peaceful?

Form 1.1 Memory and Attention Problem Record EXAMPLE

Memory and Attention Problem Record

Date: *11/1/2020* **Time:** *12* AM (PM)

How much did the memory and attention problem bother you?

0 1 2 3 4 5 (6) 7 8 9 10

Not at all Moderately Extremely

What the memory or attention problem was:

Forgot the PIN to the bankcard I was using, and I also noticed it was a different card.

What was happening (where you were, what you were doing, and what the surroundings were like, e.g., noisy, quiet, etc.)

I was in the city clerk's office, and there was a line with people talking and phones ringing, confusing!

What I felt at the time (Anxious? Tense? Hungry? Tired? Peaceful?)

Felt a little rushed as many people were waiting in line. I was also hungry since I was taking care of a chore on my lunch hour.

(words that you hear from others or from TV, radio, or online) or visual information, such as copying or transcribing telephone numbers or written materials? Alternatively, you may find that noisy environments throw off your attention or that fatigue makes it difficult to recall names. People generally vary with respect to the types of memory and attention problems they have and where and when they encounter trouble. Again, the first step in managing attention and memory problems is to improve your awareness of the situations where they are likely to arise. The next step is to target these situations and select the best strategies in this workbook to meet your particular type of memory and attention problems.

Progressive Muscle Relaxation

Another way to help with memory and attention problems is to help control the physical effects of stress. Progressive muscle relaxation (PMR) is a relaxation technique or skill that helps do this. The purpose of PMR is to help people learn to relax tense muscles and learn to better relax muscles that aren't necessary for a particular task. For instance, some people shake their leg while sitting and listening or hold a lot of tension in their shoulders. Others might find they clench their teeth while driving or grip the armrest of a chair while reading. The idea is that all that tensing takes energy and causes the nervous system to increase arousal. This increased arousal is a stress response, and this can negatively influence memory and attention. In other words, when you are relaxed, you can better focus and pay attention. And you are more likely to remember the things you pay attention to.

Becoming skilled at relaxing tense muscles takes practice. That is the downside of this exercise. On the other hand, each day, many thousands of prescriptions are written for medications that achieve the same thing. The downside of prescription medication is not only personal cost and/or side effects but also the fact that these medicines don't "teach" or "train" your nervous system to let go of tension naturally. Moreover, numerous cancer survivors who have participated in MAAT research have reported that after going through cancer treatment, they prefer not to add further medicines to their systems and would like a non-drug approach.

How It Works

Your nervous system is able to automatically run critical functions of the entire body, such as breathing, keeping the heart going to circulate blood and nutrients, and digestion, without you thinking about it. The part of the nervous system responsible for these vital functions is called the autonomic nervous system (ANS). One way to think of this is as an "auto pilot." The ANS has two branches. One activates the body and helps it escape or fight off danger when it arises. The other branch restores energy to the system and slows things down. The first branch is called the sympathetic or fight-or-flight branch. This branch activates heart rate and breathing to get vital oxygen to your large muscles so you can run away or fight off danger. This is where thinking and remembering can be affected. You don't need to solve algebra problems when you're being chased by a grizzly bear. The other branch, the parasympathetic branch, will eventually kick in once the danger has passed, and it helps restore blood flow and aid digestion. It also aids sleep; this is the branch that activates after a large holiday meal and makes us sleepy. The branches counteract each other like a seesaw (Figure 1.2).

The autonomic nervous system "seesaws" throughout our lives, each day, all day, every day. While in the 21st century we do not

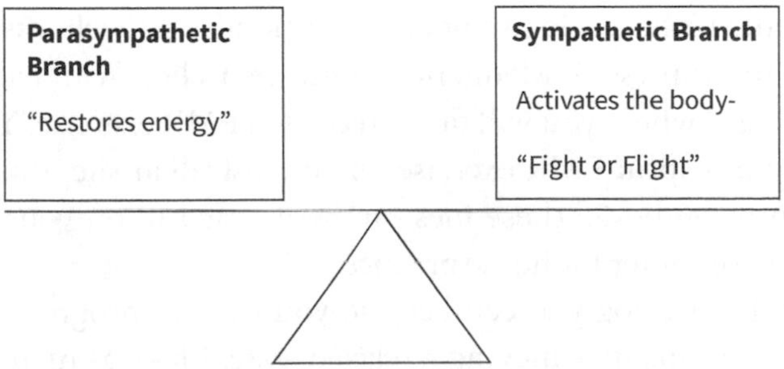

Figure 1.2 Autonomic nervous system "auto pilot."

have as many predators chasing us as our ancestors did, we retain this emergency response system, and it can create wear and tear on the body, especially if the stresses are prolonged. The key is not to avoid stress—which is impossible—but to help restore balance between the two ANS branches. One way to do this is to use relaxation techniques such as PMR. When our voluntary muscles are relaxed, we can stimulate the parasympathetic or "restoring" branch.

How To Do It

To learn to relax your muscles, you will practice a PMR exercise. The clinician will provide guidance on how to do PMR, where you will lie down and flex and relax different muscle groups, one at a time, in an exercise that will take about 15 to 20 minutes. For example, you will squeeze your right fist and gently flex the muscles of your arm for about eight seconds. Then, you will relax it. You will then move on to the other arm, then facial muscles, then legs, etc. The point of tensing and then relaxing muscle groups is to help the brain learn to let go of tension. With practice, this becomes a habit where you will let go of muscle tension almost all the time.

Your clinician or therapist may want to provide you with a practice PMR audio recording. You may also find PMR exercises that are available free of charge online. Do a simple search on "progressive muscle relaxation." Find one that suits your taste. Some people prefer music or calming nature sounds in the background, while others do not. Two suggestions are www.relaxforawhile.com or a PMR exercise found on Facebook at www.facebook/relaxforawhile. Or you may try a PMR recording at the site for student wellness at Dartmouth College. Go to students.dartmouth.edu/wellness-center, click "Mindfulness & Meditation," and then click "Guided Audio Recordings," where you will find a recorded PMR exercise. You may also find a helpful PMR exercise on an Australian site, thiswayup.org.au/pmr-audio-2. These files can be listened to on your phone, tablet, or computer for home practice.

Form 1.2 is a log you can keep so you can see progress in your practice sessions in achieving a relaxed state. Make as many copies as you like.

Form 1.2 Relaxation Practice Log

0	1	2	3	4	5	6	7	8	9	10
Not At All Relaxed					Moderately Relaxed					Very Relaxed

Date	Relaxation Level Before/After (0 to 10)	Type	Comments
___/___/__	/	☐ PMR ☐ quick	
___/___/__	/	☐ PMR ☐ quick	
___/___/__	/	☐ PMR ☐ quick	
___/___/__	/	☐ PMR ☐ quick	
___/___/__	/	☐ PMR ☐ quick	
___/___/__	/	☐ PMR ☐ quick	
___/___/__	/	☐ PMR ☐ quick	

When practicing PMR at home, keep the following tips in mind:

1) Lie as still as possible throughout your practice. If you must move, do so, but go back to lying as still as possible between flexion of muscles.
2) Do not flex any muscle until you hear the word "now."
3) Flex each muscle group at only about 30%.
4) Upon hearing the word "relax," let the muscle go completely and quickly rather than releasing the tension gradually.
5) If you have any muscle or mobility problems with any part of your body that makes tensing and relaxing painful (such as an injury or chronic pain), just focus and relax the area, without tension, or just tense the muscle gently. The point here is to become more mindful of letting tension go, not inducing pain. Let common sense prevail. (Individuals with lymphedema should check with their physical therapist or doctor to find out if gentle flexing is OK.)
6) You can use the relaxation log in Form 1.2 to keep track of your practice and progress. This isn't mandatory but can be helpful. The form has room for you to record your PMR practice and quick relaxation practice, another form of relaxation exercise you will learn in the next visit.

A Final Note on Visit 1 and Homework

You have covered a lot of ground so far. You learned about some basics of memory and attention, how cancer and cancer treatments can affect memory and attention, and how other factors such as stress, emotions, and everyday activities affect these functions. You are learning two very important memory and attention adaptation strategies already: self-awareness and stress management (Box 1.1).

If you feel overwhelmed, stop. Relax. This program is designed to go at your pace. This workbook is yours to review a little at a time, at your convenience. Write notes, use a highlighter, or do whatever it takes to help you get what you want out of it. You do not have to commit to all the exercises here. Rather, take what you need and simplify and *adapt* the useful methods to your life and your activity.

Box 1.1 Memory and Attention Adaptation Strategies in Visit 1

- Self-awareness and monitoring of memory problems
- Progressive muscle relaxation

To help you keep track of the strategies you try between sessions, a Homework Task Sheet is provided (Form 1.3). Just make a checkmark in the appropriate box for each day you do one of the tasks—note that there are 14 days, as sometimes you may not have weekly meetings and two weeks may elapse between visits. This form is simply to help you keep track of your practices and rehearsals in a quick and easy fashion. As you can see, there are many more things to learn as we go. But first, just focus on the tasks you need to complete before Visit 2: Complete some memory and attention problem records and practice your daily PMR. Review this visit in the workbook, and feel free to read ahead.

Form 1.3 Homework Task Sheet

Day: Homework Task	1	2	3	4	5	6	7	8	9	10	11	12	13	14
Assigned reading														
Self-awareness monitoring of memory and attention problems														
Self-Instructional Training														
Progressive muscle relaxation														
Quick relaxation														
Internal verbal re-hearsal strategies (SIT, rhymes, spaced re-hearsal, etc.) List here:														
External strategies (keeping a schedule, memory routine, pacing, fatigue man-agement, etc.) List here:														

Homework Task Sheet (Example)

Day: Homework Task	1	2	3	4	5	6	7	8	9	10	11	12	13	14
Assigned reading	✓	✓	✓											
Self-awareness monitoring of memory and attention problems	✓	✓	✓	✓	✓	✓	✓							
Self-Instructional Training	✓		✓	✓			✓							
Progressive muscle relaxation														
Quick relaxation														
Internal verbal rehearsal strategies (SIT, rhymes, spaced rehearsal, etc.) List here:														
External strategies (keeping a schedule, memory routine, pacing, fatigue management, etc.) List here:														

Visit 2

In This Visit You Will:

- Review your practice and response to progressive muscle relaxation.
- Learn a new relaxation skill to help keep you relaxed in daily activity.
- Review the Memory and Attention Problem Records.
- Use your recordkeeping to help you identify useful memory strategies.
- Practice the new memory and attention strategy to apply in daily life.

Homework Review

- *Progressive muscle relaxation:* If you were able to practice the PMR exercise each day, how did the practice go in general? What muscles tended to relax the most? Did you get a sense of "letting go of muscle tension"? By contrast, which muscles stayed tense?
- If you never really achieved a sense of relaxation, don't worry: The point is practice. With practice, you will *be more mindful and aware of your tension.* You'll be more aware to achieve relaxation in everyday life while catching and letting go of tension.
- If you weren't able to practice as much as you planned, ask yourself if there is anything you can change in your schedule, or whether you ready to really give this program a good try. Either way, you have taken the first steps. Before reviewing the Memory and Attention Problem Records, let's review a shorter

and perhaps more convenient relaxation exercise called quick relaxation.

Quick Relaxation

Quick relaxation is a skill that enhances your ability to quickly and effectively reduce arousal and remain calm. It involves doing brief relaxation exercises ranging from three seconds to several minutes. These quick relaxation periods are conducted dozens of times throughout the day. The idea of quick relaxation is to lower arousal before stressful events happens so that you are *optimally aroused.* That is, you are not so relaxed that you're sleepy and can't focus, but you're calmer in general. In this state, you can better focus and absorb information and may better learn it and retain it. Quick relaxation is a way to apply the effects of progressive muscle relaxation in everyday activity. Instead of waiting for the time when you listen to relaxation strategies on your smartphone or tablet, quick relaxation is designed to keep you relaxed *in the real world and in daily life.* In essence, doing many of the quick relaxation "bursts" during daily activity reminds you to stay relaxed virtually all the time. If you are mindful of maintaining optimal arousal, the inevitable stresses of everyday life can have less of a negative impact on memory and attention.

A quick relaxation exercise is done as follows:

1) First, scan your body for any tension, and focus on releasing the tension. Start at the top of your head and then focus on your neck, shoulders, arms, and each muscle down to your toes.
2) Once each muscle is more relaxed, just focus on your breathing. Do not change your breathing; just notice it. Allow your breathing to slow.
3) Each time you breathe in, say to yourself, "I am," and as you breathe out, say, "relaxed." "I am . . . ree . . . laxed." Say "relaxed" in a drawn-out manner several times. "I am . . . ree . . . laxed."

> Just continue for three or four more breaths. As you exhale, it is usually helpful to imagine that you are "blowing out" any muscle tension you may have. Do this repeatedly as long as you want, usually a few seconds to a minute or more. You may notice that you are more alert and focused.

You and your clinician will rehearse this quick relaxation exercise together, and you should try to apply this in daily life whenever you think of it, several times an hour or more. The point here is to cultivate optimal arousal and to be mindful and attentive to your state of arousal. Do this *before* demands on you increase arousal; don't wait until you need to respond to unexpected stressful events. Be proactive and apply this arousal regulation method in the real world.

Memory and Attention Problem Records: What Did You Find?

You and your clinician will review your Memory and Attention Problem Records in detail. In reviewing your records, you may find some trends. For instance, did you notice if the bothersome memory failures happened most at home, at the workplace, or in other settings? These questions can help you identify some *at-risk situations* where memory problems may be more likely to occur.

How about time of day? It may be that mornings at home involve busy routines of family members and yourself trying to get out the door to school or work. Also, cortisol is a stress hormone that gets released through the day. In the morning hours, it may enhance memory function and improve focus and recall. In the afternoon, where rising levels of cortisol may be less helpful, there may be a drop in memory function. So, time of day can influence memory. Morning may be your most focused time and when you feel sharpest (some studies suggest we are most productive with writing and learning in the morning). On the other hand, morning may be filled with noise, chaos, and feeling rushed to be on time, all of which can add to distraction and attention lapses. These questions can help identify time elements to your memory function.

Another dimension to consider is the *type of memory and attention problems* you have. For instance, are you having problems remembering spoken words, such as things others have said to you, what you heard in a lecture, or what you heard online or on the radio or TV? Alternatively, you might have problems with remembering what you read or saw (visual memory) or trouble following instruction steps. Finally, emotions, or feeling tired or hungry, may also influence all of these. When you get a good sense of some of the patterns of your bothersome memory failures, it will be easy to select the compensatory memory strategies that suit you best. For this visit, you'll be introduced to one of these strategies, Self-Instructional Training.

Memory and Attention Adaptation Strategies: Internal Strategies

The strategies in MAAT are "compensatory" in nature, meaning that each strategy is designed to prevent or reduce interference of the daily memory failures you may experience as a cancer survivor. MAAT consists of numerous adaptive or compensatory strategies, and you'll be introduced to and try a number of them. You will not use all that are listed in this workbook—you should experiment with strategies and select ones that fit your life and your circumstances. Internal strategies are behaviors you do "inside" yourself that others might not see, such as repeating a telephone number to yourself silently or using imagery or "mental pictures" to better remember someone's name. External strategies, in contrast, involve devices or cues in the environment that are external to you, such as keeping a schedule or day planner (discussed in Visit 4) or some sort of sign or note to remind you to do a task.

Internal and external strategy categories have been written about and studied by other cognitive rehabilitative experts such as Dr. Robin West[5] and Dr. Keith Ciscerone.[6] The first strategy you will be introduced to is an internal strategy called Self-Instructional Training.

Self-Instructional Training

Self-instructional training (SIT) is a strategy that helps improve your attention for completing tasks and remembering steps taken in tasks. It involves practicing "self-talk." That is, you will practice talking out loud to yourself when you are performing a task with many steps. By doing this, you become more aware of the individual steps and details, and this helps focus your attention. Research has shown this to be helpful with improving performance on many tasks for individuals who struggle with attention and short-term memory problems.

SIT involves several steps. First, your clinician will model SIT for you by talking himself or herself through a task. The task may be something you have experienced problems with, or the clinician may use the example in this workbook of filling out a form (Form 2.1). While filling out the form, the clinician might say out loud, "*Now I fill in my name on this line . . . now my address on this line*" and so forth. This is to demonstrate the strategy of self-talk by describing what they are doing.

Next, you will do the task as you talk yourself through, saying the steps out loud. You then repeat the task out loud or whisper each step. The idea is to get used to and practice self-talk in everyday, real-world situations to make your inner voice more noticeable. Eventually, you won't have to move your lips and it will become more automatic and will draw your attention to the task at hand. Repeated practice with many daily tasks can improve your focus on self-talk. Ultimately, this can improve your attention as you engage in your valued activity. By improving attention, you are more able to complete your task without missing any steps. SIT can also help improve your attention to detail. Improved attention can lead to better learning and memory storage, which means you will be more likely to recall the memory later.

Form 2.1 Practice Form for Self-Instructional Training

Today's Date____________________

Name___________________________ Date of Birth__________________

Address

____

____

____

____

Phone Numbers

Home______________________ Mobile______________________

Work_______________________

Use SIT in everyday tasks. Brewing coffee, making breakfast and cleaning up, shaving, brushing your teeth, getting dressed—all these tasks involve little steps, and many of us have been sidetracked and missed a step (for example, allowing the coffee to brew but missing the step of inserting the pot in the machine!). It's important to practice SIT with "the mundane as well as the meaningful." That is, use SIT in everyday tasks so that you will be able to use it when bigger, more important tasks come your way. Of course, SIT should be applied to tasks of high difficulty such as completing a laboratory procedure with different steps, or steps in an electrical circuit board repair, or writing software code. You be the judge.

Here is a summary of the SIT practice steps:

1) Select the practice task (or you can practice filling in Form 2.1).
2) Complete the task while talking yourself through it. Be sure to include each step.
3) If you make a mistake, simply say to yourself, "OK, I was thrown off for a second. Now, let's take the next step." Mistakes are OK; just pick up where you left off.

4) After you complete the task, repeat it—only this time, whisper to yourself.
5) After that, repeat the task again, but just silently think through each step.

Homework

Box 2.1 Memory and Attention Adaptation Strategies, Visit 2

- **Quick relaxation**
- **Self-Instructional Training**

The homework to do for your next MAAT visit is to put quick relaxation into your everyday life to optimize your stress arousal and maintain calmness (Box 2.1). Be sure to use quick relaxation often, whenever and wherever you think of it. Do not wait for stress. Instead, cultivate a level of calm, always.

Next, use SIT in everyday life. You can use Form 2.1, but practice SIT with everyday tasks, always. The more you do this "self-talk," the more automatic it will become as a way to pay careful attention. Read the section covering Visit 2 in the workbook.

Visit 3

In This Visit You Will:

- Review your practice and response to quick relaxation and your overall ability to use relaxation skills in a practical way.
- Review your use of Self-Instructional Training.
- Review any other memory and attention problems that you've noticed.
- Review strategies and select one that fits you.
- Learn how to identify and challenge thinking that leads to excessive stress or erodes your emotional strength and resilience.
- Practice the new memory and attention strategy by applying them in daily life.

Homework Review

- *Relaxation:* How well were you able to apply quick relaxation in daily life? Are you continuing to also practice the progressive muscle relaxation once per day, or several days a week? Not all methods fit all people, so you may have by now discovered some combination of relaxation exercises that works for you.
- The key here is this: Are you becoming more *mindful and aware of tense muscles and tension in daily life? And are you able to relax muscles before they build excessive tension?* Are you using relaxation to "cultivate optimal arousal" rather than waiting to get stressed and then try to wind down? With practice, this will happen.
- Obviously, too much relaxation is not what we are emphasizing here; we don't want you to be unresponsive or sleepy! But we are emphasizing maintaining an optimal level of arousal so you perform well. This is much like a track-and-field athlete. Sprinters who have too much muscle tension usually do not

run their fastest. Yes, even during a 100-meter all-out effort, world-class athletes train hours to *relax* the muscles of their upper body and jaw so that tension won't interfere with the prime objective: to move forward, fast. The aim here to keep in mind is to *relax muscles not essential for the task*. Keep up the practice you have been doing.

- *Self-Instructional Training*: Review how "self-talk" worked for you. Did it help you stay focused and on task and help you from getting sidetracked from noise such as conversations, voices, music, traffic, or other sounds? Most importantly, did you get a sense of *performing* better on daily tasks?
- Did it keep you focused visually so you weren't sidetracked by movement, objects, or reading materials? Did it help you stay focused to complete your important tasks? Did it help you avoid the temptation of glancing at email and cellphone text messages, alerts, or tweets? All of these sound and visual elements are sources of distraction.
- Remember, what you do not focus on, you will not store to memory, or you may miss a step in a task. Self-instruction (self-talk) is a helpful tool in staying "on task" and to reduce getting sidetracked. Some distractions we listed in the prior bullet are unavoidable, but some are entirely avoidable. For instance, you CAN turn off the cellphone or tablet and stow it. Minimizing distractions is discussed in "external strategies" later. For now, let's move on to more internal strategies.

Internal Strategy: Verbal and "Silent" Rehearsal

Verbal and silent rehearsal is straightforward: It simply involves repeating, silently or out loud, new information that you've just heard. The purpose of using verbal and silent rehearsal in everyday life is to improve your recall of facts, people, names, etc. Practical things may include remembering telephone numbers, addresses, or people's names so you can either recite them or write them down later.

Simple Repetition

When you hear a ZIP code, address, or name of a person you want to remember, simply repeat it out loud or silently several times, enough so you can write it down or use the information (such as dialing a phone).

Spaced Rehearsal

This is the same as verbal rehearsal but involves making the time interval slightly longer between each repetition—that is, "spacing" the intervals longer and longer between each repetition of what you're trying to remember. This method "trains" the brain to better encode or store new information. Say you want to remember a person's name. When you hear it, repeat to yourself, "Alice Jones," and then wait 3 seconds and repeat, "Alice Jones." Then wait 5 seconds and repeat, "Alice Jones," then again with an even longer interval. Visually, this would appear something like this: "Alice Jones" . . . "Alice Jones" . . . . . "Alice Jones" . . .. "Alice Jones" . . . . "Alice Jones" . . . . "Alice Jones." This method can be helpful for encoding or storing new information.

Names of People You Just Met

Forgetting the name of someone you either just met or met some time ago is quite common. It happens to many people, not only people with memory or attention problems. However, to reduce this occurrence, it is helpful to simply repeat back the name of the person you were just introduced to by looking at them, smiling, and asking to clarify if you heard the name correctly. For example, after meeting someone named Jane Jackson, you can say, "Hello. Jane Jackson? I am ________." Clarifying or repeating the person's name while looking at them helps strengthen the association between the name and the face and "deepen" the memory. You can also use this method in other social situations.

Telephone Numbers, Addresses, Etc.

Repeating back numbers either silently or out loud can help improve your memory of them, or at least help you remember until you get an opportunity to write them down. One method of helping to remember phone numbers or longer numbers is called "chunking." This involves grouping phone numbers into pairs or triplets. For example, the phone number 288-6423 can be repeated as "two eighty-eight, sixty-four, twenty-three" instead of 2-8-8-6-4-2-3. In other words, individual numbers are "chunked" into larger numbers (e.g., "6-4" becomes "64" and "2-3" becomes "23").

Whether you use verbal or silent rehearsal to remember names or numbers, daily practice and use of the strategy will yield the best results. Obviously, the best practice is when meeting new people or having someone recite a number or address to you. However, even if you have limited interactions with others, you can still practice verbal and silent rehearsal. For example, watch television news or other programs or listen to the radio and try to remember the names you hear. Also, try to remember phone numbers, addresses, or internet sites you hear on advertisements or discussed in conversation. It is sometimes a helpful exercise to memorize the mobile phone numbers of two or three of your closest loved ones rather than relying on the contacts list on your smartphone.

There are many opportunities to practice and *apply* a verbal rehearsal strategy in daily life. Do so as often as you can.

The Three Rs

Finally, a tip called the three Rs will help improve the effectiveness of silent rehearsal: Relax, Rehearse, Repeat. *Relax* your muscles and slow your breathing when listening to new information—your brain will be more receptive (quick relaxation is applicable here). *Rehearse* the new information by saying it once out loud (as in being introduced to a new person). *Repeat* the new information silently or out loud to consolidate the memory or to write it down for later use.

Rhymes

Most of us can recall nursery rhymes from childhood: "One, two, buckle my shoe . . . three, four, shut the door." The sound or "phonetic" association between similar-sounding words allows the brain to connect two bits of auditory—or word—information well. Therefore, you can use rhymes to help you remember names, numbers, or tasks to be done. The following are some examples.

Rhyming Names

This is simple with simple names, such as, "Jane from Maine," "Dan fan," "Doug on rug," etc. However, it may be a bit trickier with longer or unusual names. Don't be afraid to be creative. You may even come up with rhymes that may be unflattering to the person whose name you are trying to remember. Please don't misunderstand: We are not endorsing being cruel to others. However, adding an emotional, perhaps humorous element to the name–person association can deepen the memory and enhance its storage. For example, "Maureen the queen," "Bryant the tyrant," or "Denise has geese." Some of these rhymes may imply the opposite of their fine character or be simple nonsense, such as "Josh squash." Keep in mind that you don't have to say any of this out loud—ever!

Rhyming Tasks

A cancer survivor who was going through the MAAT program in the past indicated she had difficulty remembering the medications in her morning routine. This was critical as she also had diabetes and she needed to balance several medications to minimize complications. She came up with a rhyme that was silly but meaningful to her: "To be like Edison, take your medicine." She repeated this several times each night before going to bed as she prepared her pills for the next day. On awakening, it was nearly the first thing she said to herself.

To her, it was a commonsense verbal routine that produced greater mindfulness of taking medications.

She also reported that she often forgot to take her cup of hot coffee when she left the house each morning. As it turned out, when she did her coffee routine as the last task before leaving home, she had little trouble remembering to take the coffee with her. Her rhyme? "To have a blast, coffee last." Again, silly but meaningful to her, resulting in a smoother morning routine.

Musical Rhymes

Again, this is simple. Think of the power of advertising jingles. They stick in your mind even though it's the last thing you want cluttering up your precious consciousness. What self-respecting American does not know the Roto-Rooter jingle, or any number of Coca-Cola or McDonald's songs? The point here is this: If you want to remember a name, task, or any other concept, use rhymes and put it to song. Advertisers on Madison Avenue have known this for decades. Feel free to sing it out loud (in public, at your own risk), silently, whatever. Be creative and derive meaningfulness for yourself, so use a tune you know well.

"Cognitive Restructuring" or Challenging Unhelpful Thoughts, Beliefs, and Assumptions

"It's all about attitude." "The world is what you make it." Many people are familiar with these sayings from parents, grandparents, friends, teachers, etc. While they may seem like clichés or even annoying, there is truth to each. This section provides a brief review of what clinical psychologists refer to as "cognitive restructuring" or methods to identify, challenge, and modify automatic thoughts, beliefs, or assumptions that can erode your ability to cope effectively with stress and the strong emotions that accompany it. Cognitive restructuring is a longstanding, well-researched method used in cognitive-behavioral therapies (CBTs). It is a highly effective technique used in treatment of depression and anxiety disorders as well as coping with stress produced by many chronic illnesses, including cancer.

This section will not cover cognitive restructuring in detail, so we will keep it simple. The first thing to understand is that all human emotion comes from our rapid, microsecond thoughts or perceptions. For example, if you're lying in bed in a dark room and hear a thud in the next room, you may think, "That's a burglar!" This can lead to the emotion of fear and the fight-or-flight response discussed earlier. Your heart rate, blood pressure, and breathing increase to prepare your body for the perceived threat—this is the important *function* of anxiety: to prepare! On the other hand, you might conclude that the thud was simply the dog lying down heavily on his dog bed in the next room. In this case, the thought may produce only a minor change in emotion and trigger few if any bodily reactions.

However, when you're lying in a dark room, you can only speculate or guess what caused the thud. What do you need to do to find out for sure? Go look—gather more information. That is what cognitive restructuring is: truly examining our thoughts or assumptions to come to the most accurate conclusion so that we arrive at the most appropriate or *adaptive* emotion. Notice we don't say "right or wrong emotion." All emotions serve an important survival and adaptive function—what we need for the circumstances is the most important thing. So, if a burglar were invading, fear or anger is appropriate for escape or defensive action. By contrast, fear at that level can cause unnecessary wear and tear on the body and waste energy stores if it is only the family pet lying down to rest.

Now, of course, we offer this example only to demonstrate how your thoughts or assumptions influence your emotions. It may appear to have little relationship to what you have experienced after cancer treatment. But the influence of automatic thoughts or assumptions is powerful with respect to emotional distress regarding memory problems after chemotherapy. For instance, if you assume that a failure in memory is always due to chemotherapy, then this may lead you to overlook other, more controllable factors, such as inattention when daily memory problems arise. Considering these other, more controllable factors can lead to improved coping. The key is to know *how* to examine and challenge your thinking to enhance coping in stressful moments in cancer survivorship.

How to Examine and Challenge Maladaptive or Unhelpful Thinking

The first step in examining automatic, rapid thoughts that can produce "maladaptive" or difficult-to-manage emotion is to understand just that—they are automatic and *rapid*. Most often, we have an almost instant surge of emotion (e.g., anger, anxiety), so it may be difficult to know exactly what the triggering thought was that started the ball rolling. There are numerous methods to improve our skill at identifying and challenging maladaptive thinking, but we will focus on just two in MAAT: *realistic probability estimation* and *decatastrophizing*. Appendix 1 at the end of this workbook provides more information about identifying and challenging various types of maladaptive thinking. For a more comprehensive discussion and instruction on numerous cognitive restructuring or coping methods, see the following useful books and resources:

- *Thoughts and Feelings: Taking Control of Your Moods and Your Life* by Matthew McKay, Ph.D., Martha Davis, Ph.D., and Patrick Fanning
- *The Feeling Good Handbook* by David Burns, M.D. (www.feelinggood.com)
- Association for Behavioral and Cognitive Therapies (www.abct.org)
- *Mind over Mood: Change How You Feel by Changing the Way You Think* by Dennis Greenberger, Ph.D., and Christine A. Padesky, Ph.D.

Realistic Probabilities

Research on stress and anxiety supports the idea that when we perceive a threat, we tend to make rapid judgments about whether we have the internal and external resources to cope with (overcome) the threat. For example, when anticipating a difficult exam or test in school, how well we have prepared and the degree to which we believe we mastered the course material will determine the level of anxiety or threat we feel. Sometimes, we make snap judgments about the probability of a bad outcome without considering the realities. This snap judgment can be termed "probability overestimation." That is, we may overestimate the probability that we'll do poorly on the test.

Another example is fear of flying. According to the U.S. Federal Aviation Administration, in 2019 and early 2020 there were nearly 44,000 commercial aviation flights per day in the 5.3 million miles of U.S. air space daily (faa.gov). Most years, there are no or minimal fatal commercial aviation incidents in the United States. The real probability of dying in a commercial aviation disaster is exceedingly low. According to Dr. Arnold Barnett, a professor at Massachusetts Institute of Technology who studies air traffic operations and who at one time feared flying (see: https://www.thedailybeast.com/the-great-plane-crash-myth), the actual odds of dying in the next flight one chooses to take are about 1 in 90 million—regardless of how many times one flies (or flying every day for about the next 250,000 years). Contrast that to driving an automobile: Over a lifetime of car trips (about 50,000 per person) the odds of being killed are 1 in 140, according to the National Safety Council. Given these statistics, it is irrational to fear air travel while casually getting behind the wheel and driving down the road with no apprehension whatsoever. But many do, because they overestimate the probability of dying in a plane crash.

So how do you estimate the real probability versus the "anxious" or irrational probability? It is easy when you have numerous industry or government statistics and sophisticated databases—this is one way. But how do you challenge "anxious probabilities" in daily life? One method is to do some basic mathematical estimating.

Simply ask, "Of the last 10 times I have experienced (a situation), how many times did it result in (a negative outcome)?" Obviously 1 in 10 is 10%—or a 90% chance of a positive outcome. In short, simply ask yourself, "What is the REAL probability that (a negative outcome) will occur versus my 'anxious' probability?" With respect to memory failure, you might try challenging the thought that some disastrous consequence could occur if you forget a word during a presentation, or forget someone's name. For example, "What is the probability I will lose my job if I forget a word during my presentation? What is the real probability?" You may find the probability of the catastrophic consequence is far less than anticipated. A word of warning: If you say to yourself, "Yes, but . . ." after you examine the objective, estimated probability, you'll likely return to the original probability overestimating thought. Eliminate "yes, buts."

Decatastrophizing

We all know that the human tendency to overestimate the probability something bad might happen is one way to prepare, but too much overestimating negative outcomes leads to excessive anxiety. At the same time, exceedingly rare events can and do occur; planes do crash and people die; people do get rare diseases. Catastrophic events are possible. However, what do we do when that happens? Is it the end? No. It may certainly be the end of life familiar to us, and now that has changed. We may be shocked, mourn the loss, and then slowly, over time, learn to live with loss. We may never get over the loss (no such thing as "closure"), but we do live on with it somehow. In short, "decatastrophizing" is a form of accepting, but also understanding, that time and life events march onward. That is, while rare events can occur, we continue to live past and with these events.

A simple way to decatastrophize is to simply ask, "What then? And then what? And then what?" etc., etc. What this usually results in is the conclusion that after a negative event occurs, there is recovery and resumption of life. We learn that while we might not want to, we can adapt to circumstances and manage them appropriately.

For example, let's say you do lose your job because of cognitive difficulties leading to errors at work:

> "Then what? I would be angry, actually really scared. Then what? I would leave that job. Then what? I would reduce my spending, watch my budget. Then what? I would start calling colleagues or friends for other jobs. Then what? I would more than likely get one, because I have been offered others at this one place that likes my work. Then what? I would probably see what they could offer."

In summary, while bad things in life happen, we often avoid thinking through what we would actually do. Some clinicians theorize that painful thoughts of bad life events are too aversive, so we "stop" the catastrophic thought and distract ourselves with something else. The problem is that distraction doesn't allow full processing of the thought in a reasoned way, so once the distraction is done, the catastrophic thought with high emotion returns. In a sense, decatastrophizing helps us to confront these unpleasant life events and think through what we may *actually* do—which, quite likely, is to adapt.

In closing, another simple method of decatastrophizing is to simply say, "So?" For example:

> "I will look like a fool if I forget my supervisor's name at the meeting. So? What happens then if I do? Would I actually get fired?"

In addition, you may also conclude that the catastrophic event is so highly unlikely (low probability) that it is not even worth thinking about.

Homework

As usual with MAAT, the homework to do for the next visit is to try applying one of the verbal rehearsal strategies you think works best for you (Box 3.1). It is more important for you to master one strategy and become proficient with it than try several with no sense of mastery or practical help. Try memorizing two or three mobile phone numbers of loved ones or friends using your favorite verbal rehearsal method. Be practical.

Also, put into practice the thought challenge methods of probability estimation and decatastrophizing to any negative thoughts you may have about your memory problems. Practice them by applying them to the real world and in situations that you know may give you trouble. The more you practice, and even discuss with others, the easier and more effective it will be.

You can also use the homework task sheet seen in the Visit 1 section to keep track. In Appendix 1 there is more review of different thought-challenging methods and a written exercise. You can try this if you like. Review this section of the workbook, and if you wish you can read ahead for the next visit.

Box 3.1 Memory and Attention Adaptation Strategies, Visit 3

- Verbal and silent rehearsal
- Cognitive restructuring or challenging unhelpful thoughts, beliefs, and assumptions

Visit 4

In This Visit You Will:

- Review your practice and use of rehearsal strategies and all skills to date (relaxation, etc.).
- Be introduced to external strategies of keeping a schedule and memory routines.
- Practice the new memory and attention strategy to apply in daily life.

Homework Review

- Which methods work best for you? Is it simple verbal rehearsal, spaced rehearsal, or some combination? Does rhyming help store memory with deeper meaning, or does using melodies help? Does Self-Instructional Training have an impact or is it best used in combination with other methods?
- How about challenging maladaptive thoughts or assumptions? Does probability estimation or decatastrophizing help you cope with some of the challenges you face?
- In which situations are you most likely to use the methods? Going over these questions with your clinician will help you identify commonsense applications to improve use of your verbal working memory and attention.

External Strategies

"External strategies" refers to a set of methods that are used "outside of yourself" that may not have a direct impact on your memory and attention but can aid your memory and attention functions and avoid the pitfalls of everyday memory failures or problems associated with them.

Keeping a Schedule

The purpose of using and keeping a daily schedule is (1) to reduce the risk of becoming overwhelmed by multiple tasks and (2) to establish a regular routine to the greatest extent possible. Keeping a simplified but complete schedule can help tremendously with remembering important tasks, eliminating "to-do" lists, and freeing you from worry about missing important appointments, personal tasks, or phone calls. A good schedule is a great method of time and stress management. Surprisingly, numerous high-functioning cancer survivors do not keep an effective schedule of daily tasks. In a sense, it is as though before cancer, they did not need to keep track of personal events of work, home, and family—they were perfectly capable of keeping track of planned activity without writing it down on paper or entering it into an electronic device. However, after cancer treatment, many find that it becomes more difficult to retain and recall important events. To keep an effective daily schedule, here are suggested steps:

1) **Use a day planner.** Electronic devices such as smartphones and tablets combine communications technologies and offer a vast array of scheduling options. However, an old-fashioned paper day planner has some advantages: (1) it does not have to be charged and will not run out of battery power; (2) it requires no "set-up" time; and (3) there is no monthly fee for mobile phone or internet access. For those who like these advantages and given these upsides, buy one that has *one page for one day*. Avoid day planners with week or month displays because these do not allow enough space to write in daily tasks or appointments clearly. Conversely, hourly slots allow easy entry for tasks. Most schedules or day planners list all the daytime hours on one page, with some space devoted to evening hours:

April 5, 2021

6:00 a.m.____

7:00 a.m.____

8:00 a.m.____

9:00 a.m.____

10:00 a.m.____

11:00 a.m.____

Noon____

1:00 p.m.____

2:00 p.m.____

3:00 p.m.____

4:00 p.m.____

5:00 p.m.____

6:00 p.m.____

7:00 p.m.____

Any format close to this is useful.

2) **Write all entries in *pencil*.** Why? Because things come up in real life, and thus your schedule will need to change. Writing in pencil allows you to erase. Yes, erase—keeping a schedule forces you to see that you cannot "multitask" and do several things at once. Writing one activity in on one space helps to

accomplish this. Writing with ink will result in cross-outs and cramming in ever more information.

3) **Keep *one* schedule.** Keep a schedule for *the whole day*, not just your time at work. Activities outside of work should be scheduled, too. This includes picking up children after school or attending an evening meeting at your church or a friend's home. *Keep the schedule with you, on your person.*
4) **Eliminate "to-do lists."** A to-do list is just a list of tasks to be carried out in the future. Why not list *when* you will do each task? That is, put it in your schedule! This will likely help reduce being overly ambitious with your to-do lists and not completing what is intended. Scheduling the task forces you to schedule it when it can be done, which means it will more likely get done. If it is written in pencil, it can easily be rescheduled.
5) **Prioritize.** One problem that contributes to memory problems is scheduling too many daily tasks in addition to routine tasks. Rarely do people complete more than five or six "to-dos" over and above their normal routines. Be realistic with how much time tasks take to do.
6) **Schedule routine events first.** Block off meal times, bed times, and other routine activities to ensure routines can be established. This should be done first. Then, put in special daily events for the upcoming time period (week, month, two months, etc.). Routine events such as meals and bed times should be changed under only extraordinary circumstances.
7) **Schedule the week.** Set aside a regular Saturday or Sunday time to schedule the upcoming week. This does not have to be every activity of every day, just the highlights and important things. Do this at the same time each week (say, Sunday at 5 p.m.) to ensure it will be done and not forgotten.
8) **Use the schedule!** Make a routine where you look at the schedule before or after breakfast or at some starting point of your day. One participant in early MAAT research placed her planner in her bathroom on a shelf each night before she went to bed. In this way, she could not avoid looking at her schedule when she was done with her morning routine. Pair

your "schedule looking time" with something you already do at the start of every day.

9) **Simplify.** Keep your schedule simple. Avoid the temptation of scheduling too many tasks. If this happens, look over the schedule in the past week and schedule only those tasks that are most important and that have the greatest likelihood of getting done.

Memory Routines

Memory routines involve always doing things the same way as a regular ritual so that you don't lose things or forget the steps in a task. Examples of memory routines are:

Placing car or house keys on the same hook *every time* you walk in the door

Placing your purse to the right of the chair leg when you sit down

Keeping your day planner or electronic device in the same spot every bedtime (such as the bathroom example we just mentioned)

Having a routine for locking up your office or shop (e.g., shut off computers; check the lights, alarm, door/window locks). The *order is same each day.*

Follow these routines *without exception.*

Object placement areas are sometimes referred to as "memory places" so that you can reliably depend on the locations of objects. Examples include keeping an ID badge in the same spot on your dresser or table when it's not in use and routinely park in the same spot (or close to it).

One tip in starting a new memory place or routine is to place the object or do the task *right before or right after* doing a task you do daily now. For example, to remember the placement of an important object like your car keys, place the keys on the same hook right after walking in the door when getting home, every time. For a new task, such as taking a new daily medicine (such as hormonal therapy after breast cancer), pair taking the medicine with an existing daily task. For example, take the medicine *just before* brushing your teeth. One survivor in past MAAT research attached their toothbrush with Velcro to the medicine bottle. This was also an external cue (discussed in Visit 5) to help establish a new memory routine of taking important medicine. By doing a new task close to something you do routinely every day already, the new task will become habit.

A chart like this can help you establish new memory routines. You need not use this format, but it may be helpful in getting started:

New Object Placement/Routine	Where	When
car keys	*far left hook in mudroom*	*entering house*

Homework

Box 4.1 Memory and Attention Adaptation Strategies, Visit 4

- **Keeping a schedule**
- **Memory routines**

The homework to do for the next visit is to implement the daily schedule and try a new memory routine that can simplify your daily life (Box 4.1). As stated earlier, try any routine you think will be most useful to you. Do not feel obligated to try too many at once—one is plenty to start. The point is to do what you feel most comfortable doing and put it into daily life. Once again, you can use the homework task sheet to keep track of the methods you've used. Feel free to read ahead, but don't overwhelm yourself with new information. Simply using this workbook to review what you have learned today is perfectly fine.

Visit 5

In This Visit You Will:

- Review your practice and use of strategies and all skills to date (relaxation, etc.).
- Get introduced to more external strategies (external cueing, distraction reduction, and activity scheduling and pacing) for stress management.
- Apply the new memory and attention strategies in daily life.

Homework Review

The clinician will ask you:

- How does keeping a daily schedule simplify your life? Is your time more manageable?
- Are you looking at the schedule at set times during the day to know what's next? Are you less prone to forget important activities or appointments?
- Are you using a pencil if you have a paper day planner? Is your electronic schedule easiest in day view?
- What memory routine do you now do?
- Is it part of daily life for you?
- Can you use it in another situation?

External Cueing

External cueing is a term psychologists use for visual aids or auditory aids to remind people to do something important—in a sense, "reminders." An example of a visual cue is a sign that reads "Wash your hands before returning to work" or a green or red traffic light. An example of an auditory cue is a beep or tone that reminds you to turn off your headlights, or the ring of a phone.

External cues can help you remember to do important daily tasks such as taking medicine. For example, someone with diabetes could post a sign on the medicine cabinet that reads "1. Finger stick; 2. Blood sugar check; 3. Medication." Someone with memory problems could post a sticky note on the breakfast table that reads "look at your schedule" as a reminder to use their schedule for the day. An auditory cue such as a beeper alert on a watch or other device can be used as a reminder of a brief, scheduled work break. In short, external cues are environmental triggers of desired behavior.

Here are some suggestions for using external cues or "reminders":

1) Get a sense of your daily schedule and situations where paying attention or remembering is a problem.
2) Identify the situation, and see if a note, a sign, or an auditory reminder is best to use. If you use a sign or note, put it where you will read it, such as on the handle of the refrigerator or on a surface where there is nothing else (for instance, the seat of a chair). If you use a tone on your watch, smartphone, or desktop computer, be certain it is loud enough and different enough so it doesn't just blend into the background of other sounds.
3) Simplify. In setting up external cues, use as few words or tones, beeps, etc. as possible. Don't use too many cues; you'll just ignore the unimportant ones. One or two is best.
4) If the cues don't help remind you when to do things, change them! Make them easy, and make sure they are ones you will use. Don't be afraid to change them, especially if they are not helpful.

Distraction Reduction

In this era of electronic communications technology, there are numerous ways in which we can contact others (and they us): mobile phones, voicemail, text messaging, email, videoconferencing, social media, and other communications software. In an instant, you can get answers to questions that suddenly pop into your mind—either from others or from the banks of information available throughout the internet. But a problem arises when someone else's critical and quick need for information is not convenient to you at the moment. Say you're writing an important letter, report, or memo, you've come up with a great idea, and you're putting it into words. Just then, your cellphone interrupts you with an alert, a text message arrives, or an email window pops up, disrupting your train of thought. Then, when you go back to the task at hand, "poof!"—the working memory of that brilliant idea has disappeared.

With what some term the "creeping ivy" of electronics communication into our lives, we have, as a 21st-century culture, made ourselves available, 24/7, to anyone at any time. This is simply not possible. Yet it has become an expectation—purely a false one—of many. This intrusion into our "thinking space" has invaded not only our privacy but also our cognitive abilities. It has robbed us of deep thought and our need to have enough solitude and personal space to complete a thought and work through goal-directed tasks.

The interruptions and distractions discussed here are not trivial in terms of human attention and memory. Dr. Russell Poldrack at the University of California at Los Angeles found that when research participants were asked to complete a single task or a "dual task," they performed about the same—that is, multitasking did not result in much decline in remembering things learned during multitasking. However, brain imaging suggested that, in the dual task situation, research participants appeared to rely more on "habit learning" rather than the deeper declarative memory, or memory that is stored well and can be used in a flexible way in new situations.

This is something like learning a new vocabulary word and then using it later with a new meaning: "After the waterfall, the river is *languid* and still" and then, "A *languid* team left the field after a disappointing loss." In short, multitasking and numerous interruptions from electronic devices can lead to "incomplete" learning of new information, making it difficult to recall the information for later use or to apply it in new situations.

The growing numbers of distracted driving laws enacted nationally point to the impact these devices have on divided attention and reduced driving performance. According to data collected by the National Highway Traffic Safety Administration, in 2017 there were 3,166 distracted driving–related deaths of the 34,247 fatalities on U.S. roadways. So, while we have an abundance of information and social connectedness at our fingertips, the risks of electronic device misuse can have a public safety cost as well as causing a decline in some cognitive abilities. An interesting discussion on this topic is by Dr. Calvin Newport of Georgetown University in his book *Deep Work: Rules for Focused Success in a Distracted World*. Dr. Newport outlines how easy it is to get caught up in the distractions of mobile devices and lose the important cognitive skill of sustained attention.

We could discuss at length the negatives of these interruptions and auditory and visual distractions, but it all boils down to using some commonsense approaches to maximize your focus and concentration in learning situations. Here are some practical methods:

- *Auditory distraction.* When doing tasks that require focus, especially driving or operating dangerous tools such as saws or lawnmowers, shut off your cellphone or any other electronic devices that might interrupt you and stow them. Consider keeping the car radio off. If your vehicle has hands-free calling this may reduce the risk of distraction, but talking on the phone is still a distraction from the important task of focus on the road.
- *Work area auditory distraction.* For those who work in close proximity to others, phone conversations or personal conversations may be a distraction. Try wearing a headset (with white noise, nature sounds, or some other background sound)

or musicians' earplugs that reduce sound while still allowing important sounds (for example, your phone, your name) to get through.

- *Social setting auditory distraction.* A complaint among many chemotherapy recipients is they have a difficult time focusing on and understanding conversations with others, especially if other conversations are going on around them—such as in a small group or in a restaurant. Focus on one person at a time, and face them. Use verbal rehearsals to clarify with them what they said, or use the active listening skills discussed later in MAAT.
- *Email.* Email is one of the most abused communication devices we have. Email is not instant messaging; it is just mail. Read it once a day or twice a day at a set time (20 minutes at 8 a.m., say), and then shut it off to keep tones or windows from popping up on your computer screen. If the item someone emails you is that important, they will call. Consider setting an automatic reply on your email account that notifies people that you may not respond promptly due to the amount of email you get. Provide your phone number and instruct the reader to call if the matter is urgent.
- *Mobile phones, texting, pagers, etc.* Unless you are paid to be on call, or your family or friends may need you in an urgent manner (that is, life or death or an important deadline such as a home sale), why not turn these devices off? Texting is a highly efficient and rapid means of communication, but it is a disruption. When engaged in tasks that require your full attention, like driving, keep the device turned off, or respond only when convenient. These interruptions in attention and focus only detract from deeper memory.
- *Visual distractions.* If you get distracted by interesting or new sights, turn your workspace away from windows or doors. Face the wall, or try to arrange a walled-in space if possible. Make sure your workspace is well lit and you can see your work task easily—squinting is a form of muscle tension and can lead

to over-arousal, as seen earlier in the discusion on muscle relaxation.

Activity Scheduling and Pacing

Activity scheduling and pacing involves scheduling daily, pleasant activity to improve your mood, attention, and memory. An anxious, irritable, or depressed mood can reduce the brain's ability to focus attention. If attention is not as good as it could be, then information may be lost before it is "stored" in memory. In other words, if we can't pay attention to things, we won't be able to remember them later on.

Many cancer survivors may think, "If I'm not depressed or generally irritable or anxious, why should I bother with pleasant events scheduling?" The answer to this is a little complex but involves prevention. Identifying and doing one or two pleasant activities a day will help control stress, and controlling stress is one way to prevent anxiety, irritability, or depressed mood. As a result, this gives the brain the best chance of performing well with attention and memory. Therefore, we encourage people to schedule daily pleasant events as a way of controlling stress and maintaining or improving mood and attention. Research suggests this method can help cancer survivors improve their attention and memory problems.

Activity scheduling means scheduling any pleasant activity you wish into your daily routine. This fits nicely with keeping your daily schedule and setting realistic goals. We emphasize that activity scheduling also means *activity pacing*. Simply put, pacing means not doing too much, since overwork or excessive demands can lead to stress and then problems with attention and memory. When deciding what pleasant activities to schedule, pick simple tasks that are well within your control—for example, taking an afternoon tea break, listening to a favorite piece of music, going for a walk, exercising, or watching a favorite movie.

You can also schedule small, achievement-oriented chores like cleaning part of the bathroom or ironing a shirt—anything that is small and represents a break in routine. Chores like these may not produce the greatest amount of pleasure, but you can get a sense of achievement or satisfaction in getting a job done.

Finally, other good activities to schedule are quick relaxation breaks or the progressive muscle relaxation exercise.

Here are some suggested steps in activity scheduling. Remember to schedule activity *before* you do it. Don't wait until you are in the mood to do it. Schedule only activities you know you can do with nearly 100% confidence. The reward of a pleasant event only comes *after* the pleasant event. Remember, too, that the weather or other people can change your plans. Therefore, when planning pleasant events, you may want to include backup events in case a friend cannot meet you or the weather turns bad. In this way, you are in control of your activity—not other people or things like the weather.

Activity Scheduling Steps

1) With your schedule, you are likely familiar with your daily routine, wakeup times, mealtimes, working hours, bedtimes. Include weekdays and weekends.
2) Schedule a pleasant activity (as short or as long as desired) each day. Schedule a "backup event" in case things do not go as planned. Keep it simple.
3) Schedule some quick relaxation (as short or as long as desired), perhaps once every hour—this helps with pacing.
4) Keep track of the most pleasant or achievement-oriented events. Write in a simple 0-to-10 rating next to the event in your schedule: 0 = no pleasure or achievement; 10 = most pleasure or achievement imaginable. Remember, not all events are going to be extremes of 0 or 10 in real life; in fact, most of our activity is somewhere in the middle.

Homework

In today's visit, you learned about using external cues (or sticky notes), how to minimize distractions, and activity scheduling

Box 5.1 Memory and Attention Adaptation Strategies, Visit 5

- External cueing
- Distraction reduction
- Activity scheduling and pacing

(Box 5.1). Again, don't get overwhelmed. Just use which strategy or parts of strategies you believe are most applicable to your life. Use this workbook as your guide if you forget something. See how the methods work for you, and make modifications as necessary.

Visit 6

In This Visit You Will:

- Review your practice and use of strategies.
- Be introduced to some other strategies: active listening for following social conversation and fatigue management and sleep improvement.
- Practice the new strategies and apply in daily life.

Homework Review

- Does external cuing help you remember to complete important tasks? Is it a strategy that helps your daily life now, or is it something you may use later?
- How about the distraction reduction methods? Are you distracted more by sounds or by visual things? Both? Are you better able to focus and stay on task when you use the distraction reduction methods? What situations require distraction reduction?
- Are you using activity scheduling and pacing? Does scheduling pleasant events help with daily stress? Is pacing sensible for you?

Active Listening

This is similar to verbal rehearsal when meeting individuals and trying to remember their name (as seen in Visit 3). "Active listening" is a term psychologists and other health professionals use when describing interview behaviors. As we discussed earlier, surveys of cancer survivors who have undergone chemotherapy have found that many have difficulty following or understanding conversations when there are several small conversations going on at the same time. In fact, a sizable portion of these survivors report they avoid social activities so they don't look "stupid." Rather than avoid valuable social activities and relationships (such as valued time with friends and loved ones, book clubs, family get-togethers, community and church groups, etc.), using active listening behaviors may help improve involvement and enjoyment. If nothing else, these behaviors can help you clarify and follow conversational content. Here are the basics to try:

1) *Active Listening Behaviors.* Look at the person you are talking to. You don't need to stare or have "fixed-evil-eye" eye contact, but do face them. Keep your muscles relaxed. Convey body language that lets others know you are engaged with them.
2) *Summarization.* It is alright to summarize what you think you just heard someone say to you—not in vivid detail, but the basic gist. In short, repeat what you just heard. For example, "So you went to the store and found somc good bargains."
3) *Clarification.* This is similar to summarization but involves clarifying what you think you heard but weren't sure about. It is OK to clarify by asking a question or prefacing what you want clarified by saying something such as, "Just to be clear," "Did I hear you right?", or simply "I'm sorry, I'm a little confused. Did you say you went to the store on Maple Street and found some good bargains?"

While these active listening skills appear simple, they do take some practice so they go smoothly. The important thing is to try not to avoid situations but to use these skills assertively. All people can have difficulty focusing on conversations, lose their train of thought while speaking, and feel off track. By using these methods in daily conversations, you may be more likely to focus on the things being talked about and store them into memory so that discussion can carry on at a later time.

Fatigue Management and Sleep Improvement

Entire cognitive-behavioral treatments have been developed to improve both fatigue and sleep quality. Sleep difficulty is more common among cancer survivors than the general population, and fatigue remains a problem for many survivors even after treatment is completed. Instead of going into great detail, we will identify the basics of improving sleep quality first, and then we will outline steps to take that may help reduce daytime fatigue. For more detailed information, see the online publication "Facing Forward: Life After Cancer Treatment" at: https://www.cancer.gov/publications/patient-education/facing-forward.

Fatigue Management

Fatigue during chemotherapy is common. For some individuals it can linger for months to a year following the end of treatment, but there is no consistent pattern of fatigue across individuals, and often fatigue improves with time. The exact causes of fatigue associated with cancer treatment are unclear. Some causes may include anemia (reduced red blood cells), nutritional problems, or lack of liquids during cancer treatment, and chronic or persistent pain can make fatigue worse. Also, depression can contribute to fatigue.

Steps for Improved Fatigue Management

1) **Use the pacing methods outlined in the section on activity scheduling.** Breaking up daily tasks into smaller tasks and taking brief breaks will help prevent fatigue from building up. It is important to shift tasks at scheduled times even if you don't feel fatigued. This way, you will likely spread out your valued and busy activity over time and still achieve your goals but with better control of fatigue.
2) **Use relaxation skills.** In particular, be sure to practice quick relaxation through the day—this will help restore energy.

Again, don't wait until you are tired or run down; do this at predetermined times.

3) **Take part in sensible exercise.** Many people who have fatigue problems avoid exercise or physical activity thinking it will add to fatigue. In fact, exercise such as walking 30 minutes a day, three or four days per week, can boost energy levels, especially if you pace yourself well. As usual, before beginning any exercise, check with your doctor or health professional. If you are not sure what type of exercise to do, many medical centers have physical therapists or personal trainers in wellness programs who can make good recommendations.
4) **Diet.** Check with a dietitian to see if there are foods you should consume more of to boost energy or if there are foods to avoid that may contribute to fatigue.
5) **Medicines, supplements, or natural substances.** Check with your doctor to see if there are safe medicines that may help with fatigue. Provigil can help with daytime fatigue and may be helpful with cognitive problems. However, medicine may not be for everyone, and there may be other supplements, vitamins, or natural ingredients that can be helpful. As always, alert your health professionals about anything you are taking: although natural substances are "natural," they are not natural to your body and may interact dangerously with medicines.

Sleep Quality Improvement

Sleep is an important function for optimal health. Adequate sleep quality can boost immune system function and musculoskeletal health and help regulate mood. More pertinent to MAAT, sleep quality can boost and optimize cognitive function—memory and attention. Psychologists, neuroscientists, and other sleep researchers believe that one of the principal functions of sleep is to help the brain get its share of glucose, the sugar-based nutrient that the brain uses for energy. When you're asleep, your body is using much lower levels of glucose, allowing the brain to meet its nutrient needs and restore delicate metabolic balance. With adequate nutrition, the brain has the best chance of maintaining its memory and attention functions.

You are already practicing one method known to enhance sleep quality: progressive muscle relaxation, or the skill of keeping skeletal muscles relaxed. Continue to practice your relaxation skills and apply them to sleep—that is, when you are going to bed, let your muscles relax to the greatest extent possible.

Other steps that research has shown will improve sleep quality are discussed in the following list. The sooner you begin to implement these, the sooner you will see a difference in you sleep quality because these sleep habits will improve sleep over time. It is not as simple as taking a pill. While some medications are certainly helpful for improving sleep quality, many only initiate sleep and don't help sustain it. Further, many medications, when used repeatedly over weeks at a time, can lead to tolerance of the medication, thus requiring more to get its initial effects. Ask your primary care doctor for more information about the benefits or drawbacks of these medications.

Steps for Improved Sleep Quality

1) **The bedroom should be a "dedicated sleep chamber."** Your bedroom or sleep area should be free of wakeful distractions. This is key since the overall goal of these steps is to increase the time spent in bed asleep and not awake. Lying in bed awake only conditions the brain to be awake and promotes excessive worry about not sleeping. Avoid watching television, viewing tablets or mobile phones, or listening to music. Use the bed only for sleeping. Keep it dark when going to bed.
2) **The technology-free sleep chamber.** Blue light emitted by TV, mobile phone, tablet, and computer screens suppresses production of the hormone melatonin, the hormone that helps regulate sleep and wake circadian rhythms. Ideally, these devices should not be in the bedroom. If a mobile device is used as an alarm clock, simply keep the face of the phone downward

and ensure all audio alerts are off. Settings or apps on some devices can help promote sleep time. Try not to view devices 45 minutes prior to going to bed. In short, blue light may promote wakefulness in the way daylight might, so a technology-free sleep chamber is a good idea.

3) **Bed times, wake times.** Go to sleep and get up at the same time each day. Having a regular schedule is important to help your brain develop regular sleep stage cycles. However, remember that if you have slept fine for a few days and have trouble sleeping one night, it doesn't necessarily mean your whole cycle will get thrown off. Just continue the schedule as regularly as possible.
4) **Don't lie in bed awake for longer than 25 to 30 minutes.** If this happens, get up and go to another room. Then, do something that is relaxing (read, listen to music, or practice your relaxation skills) and return to bed when you feel sleepy.
5) **Avoid daytime napping.**
6) **Worry time.** If you find yourself habitually thinking about things in bed that produce anxiety, such as what you need to do the next day, start scheduling a few minutes during the day (not before bed) as your "worry time" or time to schedule things you need to do tomorrow. You may conclude you have done all you can that's within your control about the topic of worry, which is a resolution that will allow for the task of sleep.
7) **Wind-down time.** Remember that some people need more time to unwind before bed than others. If you need to, allow yourself an hour (or longer) to unwind before bed—take a bath, read, watch television. Never do work right up until bedtime. Always stop at least 30 minutes to an hour before bed.
8) **Caffeine use.** Avoid caffeinated beverages after 5 p.m.
9) **Exercise schedule: Keep it sensible.** Late-night exercise may be arousing and may make it difficult to fall asleep. However, regular exercise done earlier in the day can help to regulate nighttime sleep.

Homework

Box 6.1 Memory and Attention Adaptation Strategies, Visit 6

- Active listening
- Fatigue management and sleep improvement

In today's visit, you learned about using active listening behaviors to help you re-engage in social activities or focus better in social conversation (Box 6.1). You also learned about how you can use behavioral methods to improve fatigue management and sleep quality. Try one or two of these strategies. Remember, don't become overwhelmed and implement all of them at once. Do what you believe is a priority. Focus on the real-world use and application of the strategy and see how it works. Again, keep track of what you do and review this with your clinician at the next MAAT visit. Feel free to read ahead in the MAAT workbook, but don't overwhelm yourself with too much information.

Visit 7

In This Visit You Will:

- Review your practice and use of active listening and sleep strategies.
- Be introduced to visualization strategies (internal strategies).
- Tie in the strategies learned to date.
- Practice the new strategies and apply them in daily life.

Homework Review

- Are you better able to focus on conversations using active listening strategies? Does active listening help you follow one conversation at a time? More importantly, are you engaging in social activities you value, when you want to? Are you applying decatastrophizing to help you cope with small social mistakes that we all make (such as forgetting a word or name)? Is active listening helping you regain more social activity?
- Are regular bed and wake times helping you to establish a good sleep routine? Are the sleep improvement strategies helping you feel more rested when you wake up? Are you less anxious about sleep?
- Does exercise help with fatigue? Does activity pacing help with fatigue?

Visualization Strategies

Sometimes it is easiest to remember verbal information if you can get a "mental picture" of it. At its simplest, visual imagery uses mental visual pictures that are associated with a person (names), place, or thing or perhaps a task you want to remember. This is nothing new. For years advertisers have found that logos can improve sales of products when a simple visual picture becomes associated with a name. For example, what do you think of when you see golden arches along most North American highways?

Some neuropsychologists believe that by using visual imagery to remember names (places, people, objects), the brain can use circuits in the visual system to aid the auditory-verbal memory system. In a sense, the visual circuitry in the brain may be able to bypass and take over for other regions damaged or affected by cancer and cancer therapy. Some research evidence suggests that using mental pictures can improve word and name recall.

The sections that follow describe a number of visualization methods that can be helpful. You can apply these visualization methods to help you remember passwords and personal identification numbers (PIN). With all the electronic devices we have and the numerous access and security codes we need (PINs for bank accounts, passwords for online accounts, etc.), it is a wonder anyone can keep it all straight! You can also use visual imagery to commit to memory important mobile phone numbers of loved ones, just as you did with the verbal rehearsal strategy. These are just a few of the applications where visual imagery may be helpful.

Here are some methods and how to use them:

Simple Visualization

1) *State the name of what it is you want to remember.* It's always helpful to rehearse something out loud or silently if you want to remember it later. You may even repeat the name, place, or object several times. See if it sounds like something you can picture.
2) *Next, describe what you "picture" or visualize.* When you say the name, place, or object, what do you think of? For example, the word or phrase you want to remember may have a peculiar

sound association. For example, the last name Ahles—is a close association to "All-ice." You could picture a person sculpted out of ice. Or a certain place or town may already evoke a visual image—for example, a town called "MacDonald" may evoke visions of a farm or golden arches.

3) *Now exaggerate the image.* Once you think of an image associated with the word or phrase, now make it ridiculous. For example, in the "All-ice" example, you could visualize the person as a giant ice-monster looming over a city. Or picture a giant Statue of Liberty dominating the landscape. If you're trying to remember a PIN, imagine giant numbers of your PIN standing in line at an ATM. The point is that making an image exaggerated, ludicrous, and/or humorous adds to the emotional association—deeper emotion "deepens" the memory. Think of the most embarrassing moment you've ever had, your proudest moment of achievement, or where you were when you heard of the events of September 11, 2001. All have strong emotions associated with them. Therefore, create images that can evoke emotion.
4) *Visualization with a twist.* Finally, you may want to "visualize" smells with names, places, or things. Many people already can instantly identify a flower's name or the name of a spice simply by its smell but not appearance. This is also true of some towns (one author attended public schools in a rural Maine town with a large paper mill that emitted not the most flattering of odors—many people familiar with the town recall the town by its smell, not its beautiful scenery). Use smells to evoke a "mental picture" that fits the word in the same fashion as above.

The Name–Face Mnemonic ("Name–Face Association")

Many of us have trouble from time to time remembering which names go with what face. However, paying attention while looking at a person and attending to hearing their name can help consolidate a memory. An additional strategy, the name–face mnemonic, can also enhance name–face recognition. It has three steps:

1) *Think of a picture that is somehow related to a name.* For example, if you meet someone named "Brooks," you could picture a stream covered with rocks and a grassy bank. If you meet someone called "Winslow," you could associate it with "wind-slow," perhaps picturing a still sailboat adrift with flapping sails.
2) *Examine the person's face for a prominent feature.* Perhaps a nose or a forehead stands out, or their eyes, their hair, or another feature.
3) *Have the prominent feature and the image interact in some way.* Picture the visual image and the prominent feature interacting in some absurd way. For example, you could picture the stream running down Mr. or Ms. Brooks' forehead. The absurd nature of the image evokes more emotion—hopefully humor!—which helps to "deepen" the memory and will enhance the odds of later recall.

As with any verbal memory skill, practice will bring about the best results. Obviously, this strategy is best practiced in public settings where you can meet people. However, there are other ways to practice even if you have few opportunities to socialize and meet new people. Use the name–face mnemonic while watching television news broadcasts (or other programs) and practice remembering the names of the faces you see on screen. You can also practice with photos of people you see online or in magazines if their names are given in captions—anywhere a name–face association can be made. Walk away from the image and keep it pictured in your mind as you repeat the person's name. Come back in five minutes and see if you accurately recalled the name. Now walk away for seven minutes . . . and so on. Be creative in your practice methods.

Method of Loci ("The Journey")

The method of loci or "the journey" (also known as "the mental walk") is another visualization strategy to help you remember lists of words—names of objects, places, people, etc. It may be a useful way to remember a grocery or shopping list, a list of errands or "to-do" items, or new material when taking a class or academic course. It was originally used as a learning skill in ancient Greece, in the days when paper was expensive, so that speakers could remember each point they wanted to make while delivering a speech or lecture. Today, people with superior memory skills who compete in memory competitions use the method of loci.

Using the method of loci is straightforward and similar to the visualization technique we discussed earlier in this chapter.

1) *Picture a familiar space with different rooms.* This is usually done with the first floor of your home or living space, which you have walked through innumerable times. It will serve as a "visual template" in which to "place" the things you want to remember. Picture walking in the entrance you use most often and think of the path you typically follow as you walk through your home (the entryway, the kitchen, a living room to the left, a hall leading to another room, etc.).
2) *In each room, picture one of the objects or items to be remembered.* Here's where your "visual template" comes in handy. For example, we can use a simple grocery list. Picture a large gallon of milk standing in the entryway, a bag of frozen peas sitting on the counter in the kitchen, carrots standing next to the refrigerator, a ball of twine sitting in the living room, and duct tape in the hall.
3) *Once again, make the image of the objects odd or absurd.* Picture a giant gallon of milk with arms and legs and the peas spilled all over the countertop. Again, evoke emotion to "deepen" the memory. Using this type of emotional encoding or "storage method" will deepen the memory and make it easier to recall.

The most important point in using the method of loci is to use the same memory space, such as the rooms of your home, each time you want to remember a list of objects, items, or names. Most people can remember their home well, but it is the list of items or tasks that is new and most easily forgotten. Therefore, you will use the familiar space over and over again but with different objects each time you have a new set of items to remember (such as a shopping list).

If you live in a small apartment with few rooms or an open-plan house, you can use different spaces such as familiar cabinets and drawers, countertops, and closets as the memory space in the method of loci. Another alternative is using a familiar route that you use, such as your commute to work. Some individuals have used their body in the method of loci: They might visualize green beans on their head, tomatoes for a neck, milk balanced on the left shoulder, and so forth. It doesn't matter if your memory space involves rooms, a route, or body parts. The important thing is to keep it simple and to use the same memory space each time you encounter a list of things you want to commit to memory.

A final word on the method of loci: Start by remembering perhaps four rooms or spaces in which to place the objects you wish to remember. Then work up to more spaces as you become familiar with the strategy. Challenge yourself: Try running a few errands without a list. Many people use four or five rooms to remember lists of about that length and then work up to more items. As with anything, practice and daily application will make the strategy simple and easy to use with time, so commit the time to mastering the method.

Homework

In today's visit, you learned about using visualization strategies to pair visual information with other sensory experience (auditory) to improve memory storage and later recall (Box 7.1). Try one or two of these strategies. Once again, keep it simple. Don't become

Box 7.1 Memory and Attention Adaptation Strategies, Visit 7

- Visualization strategies

overwhelmed and implement everything at once. Do what you believe works best and is practical for you. Apply these strategies in daily life and see how it works. Again, keep track of what you do and review this with your clinician at the next visit.

Visit 8

In This Visit You Will:

- Review your practice and use of visualization strategies.
- Tie together strategies learned to date.
- Maintain strategies learned and adapt them to future changes.
- Discussion and wrap-up.

Homework Review

- Are you using visualization strategies to help you recall things?
- Are you using them to help you recall names of people you have recently met? How about passwords or personal identification numbers (PINs) for bank accounts, daily tasks or running errands without a list, or any number of similar applications?
- How are you using other strategies at the same time, such as relaxation skills, verbal rehearsal strategies, and using a schedule (day planner)?

Tying Together Strategies and Maintenance

To date, you have learned a number of strategies to help you compensate for and self-manage memory and attention problems related to cancer. These strategies have combined methods that are internal (ones you can use in your mind or with your voice) and external (strategies using devices such as a daily schedule). You have also learned and applied some basic stress management strategies: applied relaxation skills and activity pacing and scheduling. Table 8.1 summarizes all these strategies.

Table 8.1 MAAT Strategies

Visit 1
- Self-awareness and monitoring of memory problems
- Progressive muscle relaxation

Visit 2
- Quick relaxation
- Self-Instructional Training

Visit 3
- Verbal and silent rehearsal
- Cognitive restructuring or challenging unhelpful thoughts, beliefs, and assumptions

Visit 4
- Keeping a schedule
- Memory routines

Visit 5
- External cueing
- Distraction reduction
- Activity scheduling and pacing

Visit 6
- Active listening
- Fatigue management and sleep improvement

Visit 7
- Visualization strategies

Now that you have learned skills for managing memory and attention problems, the key is to maintain the new behaviors that you have worked hard on acquiring. Research on health behavior change suggests that it takes a number of weeks of daily practice until a new behavior becomes routine. The main points here are:

1) By practicing good memory and attention habits (MAAT strategies), memory and attention failures can be prevented, or, when they do arise, will be better managed.
2) Memory problems are to be expected, particularly in times of increased stress or when upsetting life events occur. The skills

you learned in this program will be most useful when memory difficulties arise.

3) However, an important point is to practice the attention and memory strategies presented in this workbook *on a daily basis.* Do NOT wait until memory and attention problems arise. Once you begin regular use of the skills you learned here to cope with and manage symptoms, dealing with them becomes automatic and natural.

A maintenance plan for maintaining your skills should include the following five points: self-evaluation, the importance of pacing, the importance of practice, review, and the importance of social support.

Point 1: Self-Evaluation

At least once a month, use the Memory and Attention Problem Record for two or three days in a row. You can make additional copies as needed. The reason for this is to look closely at what situations contribute to what types of attention and memory problems. See if the 0-to-10 ratings are lower or higher, and note if stress has an effect on attention and memory. By writing it down, you can take a careful look at what the problem situations are—such as at work or when you are tired—and identify the most effective skills that can help. As life circumstances change (as they do for all of us), we may face different memory demands. Therefore, this self-assessment can be helpful in determining what life changes have taken place and whether they demand different memory skills.

For example, a nurse may have a job that mostly involves administering intravenous (IV) medications. The nurse may use Self-Instructional Training skills to make sure no steps in the administration process are skipped and no errors are made during IV medication administration. But if the nurse takes a new job that mostly involves conducting educational sessions, such as in a diabetes service, more verbal rehearsal and active listening skills will be important to recall names and teaching points.

Point 2: The Importance of Pacing

If you notice you are increasingly tired or fatigued, you might want to devote more attention to good activity pacing. Activity scheduling and pacing can help with fatigue management, as can the relaxation skills you have learned.

Point 3: The Importance of Practice

Using the most valued strategies in this workbook every day is practice. You are encouraged to refine and apply other strategies in addition to the ones (at least two) you are applying every day. However, keep it simple and emphasize the practical.

Point 4: Review

At least once a month, look over this workbook to refresh your understanding of the skills that are most helpful and important to you. Also, look over the other portions of the workbook so that you don't miss information that could be helpful to you. Again, your life circumstances may change with a move, new job, or family circumstances. You thus may have new tasks, routines, or job demands that require different forms of memory. Therefore, strategies that you may not find useful at present may become useful in the future. This monthly review can help you be prepared for such change.

Point 5: The Importance of Social Support

Health psychologists have long known that having regular interaction with loved ones, friends, spouses, neighbors, family, co-workers, or close others can boost many aspects of health. "Social support" has been demonstrated to boost some immune system functions and is associated with longevity. It has also been demonstrated that social support can help people cope with the burden of cancer and maintain new health behaviors. This does not mean you have to have a large network of friends or throngs of admiring community members or fan clubs. You don't have to be the life of the party. Rather, if you are satisfied with the quality of supportive others in your life who have helped you through cancer or other health challenges, or life in general, this would qualify as good social support. To help you maintain the new strategies you have learned with MAAT, talk to your social support network and ask them to help you keep on track. For example, ask them to quiz you to help you remember names or directions and to play games that require memory, vocabulary, and reasoning skills. Take a course together. Try to schedule regular exercise together. You may even share this workbook with your social support network and commit to using strategies together daily, such as use of a daily schedule, activity scheduling, or daily progressive muscle relaxation. In short, social support has many health benefits and often it is cost effective (that is, inexpensive). The key is to reach out and ask—you may also be giving something in return.

Form 8.1 is a written maintenance plan. The point of the form is to have a written plan for maintaining behavioral skills on your own. You should complete this with your clinician. Keep in mind that the point of this plan is to help you keep up with your memory and attention skills always.

The End of the Beginning

As a cognitive-behavioral program, MAAT has covered a lot of material. You have learned about the various effects different forms of cancer and cancer treatments can have on memory and attention and the typical types of memory problems experienced by many individuals who have never had cancer treatments. You have also learned and applied a variety of adaptive strategies to help you improve performance in daily life *where you use your memory*. This is now "the end of the beginning," and now you will begin to refine,

Form 8.1 Maintenance Plan

1. In the table below, list the adaptation strategies you prefer and use most in the left column. In the right column, indicate if you use the strategy daily and under what situations you are likely to use it (for example, work, home, or community). Review this once per month. Revise as needed.

Strategy	When Used, How Often? What Situations?

2. What day and time will you review your MAAT workbook each month?

3. Social support: Who will you use to help you keep on track? When will you use or ask your social support network for help?

reuse, and find creative ways to apply all the MAAT strategies for improving memory function in your daily life.

This visit does not have to be your last contact with the clinician you are seeing. You may, from time to time, if your health or life circumstances change or other factors arise that affect daily memory function, re-consult your clinician for two or three visits for a "booster." This may not be necessary, but in some cases it may be useful. For now, continue with the new strategies and refine their application.

References

1. Miller KD, Siegel RL, Lin CC, Mariotto AB, Kramer JL, Rowland JH, Stein KD, Alteri R, Jemal A. Cancer treatment and survivorship statistics, 2016. *CA Cancer J Clin.* 2016;66(4):271–89.
2. Siegel RL, Miller KD, Jemal A. Cancer statistics, 2020. *CA Cancer J Clin.* 2020;70(1):7–30.
3. McDonald BC, Conroy SK, Ahles TA, West JD, Saykin AJ. Alterations in brain activation during working memory processing associated with breast cancer and treatment: A prospective functional magnetic resonance imaging study. *J Clin Oncol.* 2012;30(20):2500.
4. Kesler SR, Kent JS, O'Hara R. Prefrontal cortex and executive function impairments in primary breast cancer. *Arch Neurol.* 2011;68(11):1447–53.
5. West R. *Memory fitness over 40*. Triad Publishing; 1985.
6. Cicerone KD, Dahlberg C, Malec JF, Langenbahn DM, Felicetti T, Kneipp S, Ellmo W, Kalmar K, Giacino JT, Harley JP, Laatsch L, Morse PA, Catanese J. Evidence-based cognitive rehabilitation: Updated review of the literature from 1998 through 2002. *Arch Phys Med Rehab.* 2005;86(8):1681–92.

Internet Resources

American Cancer Society:
(https://www.cancer.org/treatment/treatments-and-side-effects/physical-side-effects/changes-in-mood-or-thinking.html)

National Cancer Institute: "Facing Forward: Life After Cancer Treatment" (https://www.cancer.gov/publications/patient-education/facing-forward)

References

[illegible]

Internet Resources

[illegible]

APPENDIX 1

More on Changing Maladaptive/ Unhelpful Thinking

This appendix gives a list of "maladaptive thinking styles." This list is seen in various forms in the cognitive-behavioral resources listed in the Visit 3 section. Most of us from time to time engage in these styles of thinking, which can produce strong stress responses and emotions when big life challenges come along. We are only human, so don't view each category as "right or wrong" thinking. However, each can lead to overreactions of emotional distress and defeat positive coping. Probability overestimation and catastrophizing, covered in the Visit 3 section, are listed first, but there are many other styles of thinking that can lead to more emotional distress. Which ones do you recognize in yourself? Note that some may overlap, such as "black or white" thinking with "overgeneralization" or "mental filter" and "disqualifying the positive."

Maladaptive Thinking Styles

1) **Probability Overestimation:** Overestimating the probability that a negative outcome will occur. For example, many fears or phobias are associated with overestimating risk or danger (e.g., fear of flying or injections).
2) **Catastrophizing:** Thinking the worst and believing that one will not or cannot cope with a negative event. Example: "Not getting that job will be the worst thing that could happen to me!"
3) **All-or-Nothing Thinking:** Also known as black-or-white thinking. Examples: "If I'm not perfect, I'm a failure" and "99% right is 100% wrong."

4) **Overgeneralization:** Seeing one negative event as a never-ending pattern.
5) **Mental Filter:** Unable to think of anything but one negative detail. One minor flaw ruins the whole thing (or day, event, etc.).
6) **Disqualifying the Positive:** Positive experiences don't count. Negative beliefs are maintained even when they're contradicted by experience or available evidence to the contrary.
7) **Jumping to Conclusions:** Making negative interpretations even when there are no facts to support a given conclusion. Two types:
   A. *Mind Reading*: Concluding that someone is reacting negatively to you without bothering to check it out.
   B. *Fortune Telling*: Anticipating that things will go badly, and becoming convinced that your prediction is an already established fact.
8) **Magnification or Minimization:** Exaggerating the importance of things (e.g., your mistake or someone else's achievement) or reducing the importance of other things (e.g., your own positive qualities or another person's imperfections).
9) **Emotional Reasoning:** Assuming negative emotions reflect the way things really are. Examples: "I feel it, so therefore it must be true" and "I feel this is dangerous, and therefore it must be so."
10) **"Should" Statements:** "Should" statements imply a rule that cannot be violated. While life is full of rules, sometimes they are self-imposed and do not reflect reality. Examples: "I *should* be able to do this without mistakes" and "People *should* always say please" (do they?).
11) **Labeling and Mislabeling:** Extreme form of overgeneralization; for instance, instead of describing your mistake, you label yourself a "loser." Language is usually highly colored and emotionally loaded.
12) **Personalization:** Seeing yourself as the cause of an external negative event for which you were not primarily responsible, or believing you are the cause of some negative event or someone's displeasure or unhappiness when there is little to no evidence.

Changing Maladaptive Thinking

Try using the following four-column chart. It is similar to the self-awareness methods you used earlier to better understand daily memory problems. This exercise helps to "slow down" the thought process and catch maladaptive thoughts so they can be examined and challenged. Once a day for about a week or so, complete one of these forms at the end of your day. It's even better to complete the form as soon after an emotional experience as possible, but this may not always be convenient.

In the far-left column labeled "emotion," write down a stressful or negative emotion you had during an experience that day (frustration, anger, annoyance, etc.). You may want to limit your experiences to problems with memory or attention, but that is not necessary. Next, indicate the level of intensity of the feeling using the 0-to-10 scale provided. In the next column, try to recall exactly what you were thinking at the moment you first had the emotion. Don't worry about being perfect. Just give your best guess as to what you thought.

Next, use the list of maladaptive thinking styles to try to identify which category of thinking style could apply (see column labeled "Type of Maladaptive Thinking"). Finally, in the column to the far right, come up with alternative thoughts that challenge the maladaptive thinking. Be honest, but try to really challenge the thinking that is triggering the distressing thoughts—if you don't, you'll simply maintain status quo thinking that leads to status quo distress. See the sample of this exercise provided.

Maladaptive Thought Modification Record

Emotion Rate: 0 = Nothing 10 = Worst	**Automatic Thought**	**Type of Maladaptive Thinking**	**Rational or Coping Thought**
Frustration! 6	Here is my chemofog again! I *always* forget names—it is the worst thing that can happen to me!	Using absolutes (the word "always"); catastrophizing	OK, it is frustrating, but I don't *always* forget names; sometimes I do, and it is usually when I'm a bit rushed. No, it is *not* the worst thing that can happen. It is frustrating, but not the worst thing—I've been through much worse!

Maladaptive Thought Modification Record

Emotion	Automatic Thought	Type of Maladaptive Thinking	Rational or Coping Thought

Index

Tables and figures are indicated by *t* and *f* following the page number